Chesneys' Care of the Patient in Diagnostic Radiography

Other books of interest:

CHESNEYS' EQUIPMENT FOR STUDENT RADIOGRAPHERS
Fourth Edition
Edited by P.H. Carter
with A.M. Patterson, M.L. Thornton, A.P. Hyatt, A. Milne, J.R. Pirrie
0-632-02724-X

RADIOGRAPHIC IMAGING
Fifth Edition
Edited by John Ball and Tony Price
0-632-01943-3

ESSENTIAL PHYSICS FOR RADIOGRAPHERS
Second Edition
J.L. Ball and A.D. Moore
0-632-01482-2

MRI IN PRACTICE
Catherine Westbrook and Carolyn Kaut
0-632-03587-0

HANDBOOK OF MRI TECHNIQUE
Catherine Westbrook
0-632-03884-5

REVIEW QUESTIONS FOR MRI
Carolyn Kaut and William Faulkner
0-632-03905-1

Chesneys' Care of the Patient in Diagnostic Radiography

Seventh Edition

Pauline J. Culmer

MSc, TDCR, PGDip, MIMgt, MIPD
Head of Department and Course Director
Department of Radiography Education
University of Wales, Bangor

Blackwell
Science

© 1962, 1966, 1970, 1972, 1977, 1986, 1995 by
Blackwell Science Ltd
Editorial Offices:
Osney Mead, Oxford OX2 0EL
25 John Street, London WC1N 2BL
23 Ainslie Place, Edinburgh EH3 6AJ
238 Main Street, Cambridge,
  Massachusetts 02142, USA
54 University Street, Carlton,
  Victoria 3053, Australia

Other Editorial Offices:
Arnette Blackwell SA
1, rue de Lille, 75007 Paris
France

Blackwell Wissenschafts-Verlag GmbH
Kurfürstendamm 57
10707 Berlin, Germany

Blackwell MZV
Feldgasse 13, A-1238 Wien
Austria

First published 1962
Second edition 1966
Third edition 1970
Fourth edition 1972
Reprinted 1974
Fifth edition 1977
Reprinted 1979, 1982
Sixth edition 1986
German translation 1970
Seventh edition 1995

Set by DP Photosetting, Aylesbury, Bucks
Printed and bound in Great Britain at
the Alden Press Limited, Oxford and Northampton

DISTRIBUTORS
  Marston Book Services Ltd
  PO Box 87
  Oxford OX2 0DT
  (Orders: Tel: 01865 791155
          Fax: 01865 791927
          Telex: 837515)

North America
  Blackwell Science, Inc.
  238 Main Street
  Cambridge, MA 02142
  (Orders: Tel: 800 215-1000
                617 876-7000
          Fax: 617 492-5263)

Australia
  Blackwell Science Pty Ltd
  54 University Street,
  Carlton, Victoria 3053
  (Orders: Tel: 03 347-5552)

A catalogue record for this book is
available from the British Library

ISBN 0-632-03762-8

Library of Congress
Cataloging in Publication Data
Culmer, Pauline J.
    Chesneys' care of the patient in diagnostic
radiography.—7th ed./Pauline J. Culmer.
      p.   cm.
    Rev. ed. of: Care of the patient in diagnostic
radiography/D. Noreen Chesney, Muriel
O. Chesney. 6th ed. 1986.
    Includes bibliographical references and index.
    ISBN 0-632-03762-8
    1. Radiography, Medical.   2. Nursing.
3. Radiologic technologists.   I. Chesney,
D. Noreen. Care of the patient in diagnostic
radiography.   II. Title   III. Title: Care of the
patient in diagnostic radiography.
    [DNLM: 1. Radiography.   2. Nursing Care.
WN 200 C9674c 1995]
RC78.C459   1995
616.07′572—dc20
DNLM/DLC
for Library of Congress   94-30883
                                                CIP

*Dedicated to those colleagues who have assisted me during the process,
to the students who have provided the inspiration to persevere and
to my husband who has been so understanding.*

Contents

Preface to Seventh Edition

Care of the Patient in Diagnostic Radiography was the first textbook I bought right at the beginning of my student training. I remember reading the descriptions of barium enemas with a fascinated horror and wondering exactly what I had let myself in for. The book has remained a standard text and whilst there are other books, both in radiography and nursing which cover the same field, there are none, I believe, which do so quite as comprehensively as this one. It was therefore with great enthusiasm (but also with trepidation) that I committed myself to producing a seventh edition.

I have tried to preserve the flavour of the Chesneys' writing but at the same time to provide a textbook for radiography education in the 1990s and beyond. In the UK this is now at degree level and this book attempts therefore to document some appropriate research and to encourage the student to read further about each topic from journal articles, relevant legislation and other standard texts. Chapter 1 also attempts to set the context of patient care at a conceptual level which is currently fairly unique in radiography, using research of my own which is ongoing.

The *need* to read around this subject has never been greater; many of the subjects covered merit in-depth research in their own right. In particular, the study of behavioural science is now generally taught in radiography as a separate discipline and as such is not treated in this text in any depth. Some may feel this opens the book to criticism, but I feel it is an appropriate reflection of current educational thinking. The book includes substantial revisions in the light of recent legislation, for example in Chapter 2 on transfer techniques. Certain aspects of patient care have been relocated so that the information is now to be found in the chapter covering the system/tract to which it relates. Hopefully this has made the order of contents easier to follow.

I would like to acknowledge the assistance of those who have given me specific help in the preparation of the book: Mary Wright, Gemma Halligan, Amanda Marr, Craig McKillop, Veronica O'Neill and the staff at Ysbyty Gwynnedd in Bangor for posing for the new photographs; Andrew Shaughnessy for the photography and other help with the text; Elaine Nattress, Jill Newman and Helen Hughes, all from the Maelor Hospital, Wrexham who helped me with various chapters; the Medical Art Department at the Royal Marsden for illustrations; Jacky Arrowsmith for allowing me to pick her brain at various stages and my other colleagues in the School in Wrexham for supporting me during the project.

Pauline Culmer
Summer 1994

Preface to First Edition

This book has been written because there seemed to be a need for it. Care of patients in the X-ray department has long been a responsibility accepted by radiographers, and it is possible that a textbook on the subject is overdue. Now recent changes in the syllabus of training and the examinations for the Diploma of Membership of the Society of Radiographers have made it necessary for students to receive formal instruction in this aspect of their work. We hope that this book will be of some help to them, and perhaps also to their teachers.

At the same time we have not felt that this section of the syllabus of training should rigidly define the boundaries of the book, and we know that we have included more detail than is likely to be required by the student preparing for Part I of the MSR examination. We hope that senior students and perhaps also some radiographers may find it of value.

We are pleased to find opportunity here to express thanks to those who have given us assistance. In particular we are grateful to our always helpful consultant radiologists at the General Hospital, Birmingham, and at the Coventry and Warwickshire Hospital, Coventry. Dr J.C. Bishop, Dr J.E. Glasgow, Dr J.B. Hearn, Dr J.F.K. Hutton, Dr P. Jacobs and Dr G.A. Macdonald were good enough to read various parts of the manuscript, and between them covered Chapters 1 to 11 and Chapters 13 to 17. We are indebted to them for the gift of their time and interest, for their helpful and detailed comments, and for the encouragement with which they sustained us. Mr R.F. Farr, Chief Physicist at the Department of Physics of the United Birmingham Hospitals, was kind enough to read Chapter 20 and a section of Chapter 18, and gave us the help of his comments. We are grateful to Dr F.G.M. Ross of the United Bristol Hospitals for a personal communication in connection with spleno-portal venography. Photography was undertaken by Mr T.F. Dee of the Department of Medical Photography at the Queen Elizabeth Hospital, Birmingham. We are glad to express our thanks to him, and to Miss W.L. Brookman, Superintendent Radiographer of the Radiodiagnostic Department, to members of her staff, to student radiographers, and to a patient for co-operation and help willingly given for these photographic illustrations. For the bulk of the remaining illustrations we are grateful to the following for the loan of blocks and art material and permission to reproduce in publication: Baillière, Tindall & Cox Ltd; Bowater-Scott Corporation Ltd; Messrs A.C. Cossor & Son (Surgical) Ltd; Down Bros. and Mayer & Phelps Ltd; J.G. Franklin & Sons Ltd; The Genito-Urinary Manufacturing Co. Ltd; Macarthy's (Wholesale Chemists) Ltd; Her Majesty's Stationery Office; Charles F. Thackray Ltd; and Watson & Sons (Electro-Medical) Ltd.

Lastly, or perhaps firstly, we wish to thank Mr Per Saugman of Blackwell Science Ltd for being always so helpful and for beginning it all.

D. Noreen Chesney
Muriel O. Chesney

Chapter 1
Patient Care and the Radiographic Process

Introduction

The very first statement in the previous edition of this book was that 'care of the patient in radiography is not a static subject' (Chesney & Chesney, 1986). It is certainly true to say that in the years since that statement was made, there have been many changes in the profession as a whole and in the education of student radiographers. Those students who read this edition will (in the UK certainly) be without exception reading for a degree in radiography. This new edition therefore attempts to reflect that major educational change by the inclusion of references and new information as appropriate. This chapter introduces two conceptual models of the radiographic process and outlines how these frameworks might guide the whole approach to patient care in diagnostic radiography.

The health continuum

A number of authors have postulated in different ways that there exists a health–illness continuum. Castle (1988) suggests that this continuum represents two different approaches to health care: at one end there is the medical profession whose aim is to 'treat illness' and at the other end of the continuum lies a more social (or holistic) model which is embraced by nursing and other paramedical professions and has as its starting aim to 'promote health'. Castle stated that the profession of diagnostic radiography lay more towards the medical end of the spectrum owing to its pre-occupation with the signs and symptoms of illness and the tendency of radiographers as a whole to refer to patients by their component parts or in terms of the examination they are about to undergo ('I've just done a hand'; 'Has that barium meal arrived yet?'). Castle proposed that as time went on there would be a move towards a more holistic perspective, prompted in part by the introduction of behavioural science teaching into undergraduate training courses. The study of psychology aids in the understanding of patients' reactions to disease and to the examinations which are inflicted

1

upon them. The study of sociology allows us to understand why there are inequalities in health, and the factors which impact upon people's health and well-being.

Torres (1989), p. 7, took a different view of the health–illness continuum and stated that the health of any individual can be placed on a line whereby:

> 'At the positive end of the continuum, all body organs are in top working function with one's mental faculties working at their best. At the negative end, a person is close to death or despair. In the middle are persons in all states of mental and physical well-being ranging from good health to illness . . .'

> (Torres, 1989)

Roper *et al.* (1980) use a similar concept by describing a dependence–independence continuum. At any point in the lifespan according to age and physiological or mental state a person may be relatively independent or very dependent upon others for any or all aspects of their care.

It is certainly the case that in any department of medical imaging there will be patients who may be at completely opposite poles of the continuum or at any point in between. Our patients may be very young or very old, they may be seriously ill or not ill at all and may be coming for some form of screening procedure or because they are pregnant (McClellan, 1990).

The radiographic process

As stated in the introduction to this chapter, it is the intention to introduce two models which attempt to depict the radiographic process. The models are the initial product of research which is still in progress and as the research continues it is likely that they will be modified over time (Culmer, 1994). They are therefore introduced on that basis, but it is felt that even at this early stage in the research the models provide a useful spur to the discussion of patient care in diagnostic radiography. The initial idea for the research came from my experiences of being a clinical tutor. Students will probably be aware that it is comparatively easy to learn to radiograph patients' hands and feet and to carry out other skeletal examinations on fit healthy adult patients. The complexity and degree of difficulty of examinations comes with patients who are closer to the dependence end of the continuum described by Roper *et al.* (1980). In order to examine such patients it is no longer possible to rely solely on the textbooks for our techniques; there is a need to apply higher order skills in order to successfully carry out the examination required.

Methodology

The early stages of the research were carried out using inductive methodology. Groups of radiographers and students were asked about the process by which they would examine a patient who had been sent round from the Accident and Emergency Department on a trolley. They were to imagine that the patient had multiple injuries and that the request was for a range of projections. The first stage was that the groups were asked to write down words or phrases which would describe the radiography of such a patient. When they had done this they were asked to use the words and phrases to draw a diagram of the process itself. This stage yielded two models broadly similar to Figs. 1.1 and 1.2. About 60% of respondents produced a diagram which roughly corresponded to Fig. 1.1. and the remaining 40% produced diagrams which corresponded in some way to the shape of Fig. 1.2. The words which are used to characterize the stages of the models were drawn initially from the words and phrases which were produced by the groups. At

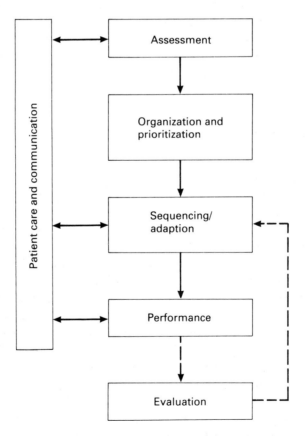

Fig. 1.1 Linear model of radiographic process.

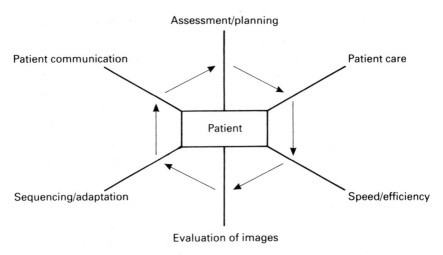

Fig. 1.2 Subsidiary (holistic) model of the radiographic process.

a slightly later stage these words were put into a list of the 25 most common which the groups had used. A subsequent sample of over 50 radiographers was then given the list in the form of a questionnaire and asked to rate their importance as part of the process of radiography of a trauma patient. The models as shown in Figs. 1.1 and 1.2 have been modified from the responses to that questionnaire. Let us then analyse the two models that have been produced.

Model 1 – linear

Stage 1 – Assessment

The first part of the radiographic process commences with an assessment of the patient and the examination to be carried out. This assessment may start before we even have sight of the patient. The request card comes down to the department; depending upon the circumstances this may well be in advance of the patient attending the department. If the card comes down from the ward, for example, the radiographer assesses the patient's clinical history and associated information. Can the patient come down in a chair? Does the examination require a special room in the department? Does the examination requested need the services of a radiologist? Is the request for a mobile examination? All of these questions need to be assessed and only then can the radiographer schedule the patient's examination. This process may require liaison with different departments in the hospital – for example the ward itself or the portering department. Some patients may require the assistance of the ambulance service in order to attend for their examination.

Thus the radiographer begins to interact with other health care workers as part of a multidisciplinary team.

Once all this has been arranged and the patient arrives in the X-ray department a further assessment process takes place. The particular capabilities of the patient must be assessed before the examination commences. Can the patient stand or get onto the table unaided? Is the patient conscious and/or co-operative? Does the patient have a condition which may render them unable to keep still during the examination? All of these points must be considered by the radiographer before commencing the examination.

Stage 2 – Organization and prioritization

Even examinations which seem relatively uncomplicated require some organization on the part of the radiographer. Based upon the assessment of the patient's condition the projections are arranged into an order of priority (Fig. 1.3). It is a principle of radiography to undertake first those projections which may seem to be easier for the patient to adopt. In this way we attempt to ensure the patient's co-operation for subsequent projections which may be more painful or more difficult for the patient to achieve. With certain categories of patients the projections are also prioritized such that the minimum amount of movement is required on the part of the patient. Thus all seated projections may be undertaken on an elderly patient before the patient is moved onto the X-ray table.

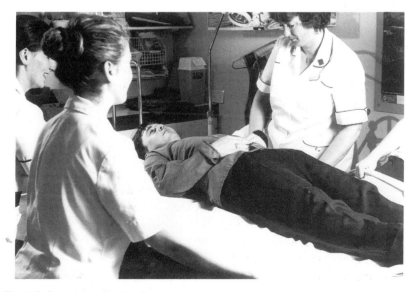

Fig. 1.3 Organization and patient assessment.

Alongside this process of prioritization of projections, the radiographer has other elements of the examination to organize. The room must be set up beforehand, with all necessary equipment to hand, so that the patient's actual examination time is minimized. The availability of previous cards, reports and films must be checked so that unnecessary projections (and thus radiation exposure) are avoided.

Stage 3 – Sequencing and adaptation

Throughout the examination the radiographer must be aware of the patient's condition so that where necessary the sequence of the examination can be modified. For example, if a patient becomes dizzy or weak during the procedure then projections which might otherwise have been undertaken with the patient standing will be carried out seated; anteroposterior instead of posteroanterior etc. Projections may also be modified to take into account the patient's abilities to attain certain positions. A prime principle of radiography is to obtain two views at right angles to each other. For patients who are badly injured these may not be the standard projections. A simpler example would be the use of the posteroanterior projection of the thumb instead of the anteroposterior, which can be difficult and painful to achieve. The sequencing of projections may be modified after initial films have been evaluated, to include further views where required; oblique projections, for example.

Patient care and communication

All these three stages plus the performance of the examination itself require constant patient communication and care for the patient throughout the radiographic process. This is the main subject of this book. The dangers of overemphasis on the technical aspects of radiography to the detriment of effective patient care have been commented on elsewhere (Makely, 1990). It is only by constant communication with the patient throughout the examination that the radiographer is able to assess their condition and adapt the examination so as to provide the best care for the patient whilst achieving a technically excellent image. As Dwane (1993) reminds us, the end product of a radiographic examination should include '... a happy, comfortable patient who leaves the department feeling she has been treated well and who remembers the experience as something good and positive.' Dwane also comments on the need to make time to care for patients and the temptation to brand some patients as 'difficult'. Ehrlich & McCloskey summarize the public's expectations of how a professional should behave:

'The best radiographers love their work and their patients. They treat patients with the same kind of concern that they would appreciate if they were ill. They realize that some people are rigid and intolerant, especially when feeling anxious.'

(Ehrlich & McCloskey, 1989, p. 27)

Stage 4 – performance

During the performance of the examination attention to the patient's condition through constant observation and communication are critical, both from the point of view of general patient care but also with regard to the health and safety of the patient. A patient who is feeling faint, for example, may fall and injure themselves. A sudden deterioration in the patient's condition may require medical help to be summoned, or more simply may need further adaptation of the radiographic techniques used. Pressure on resources may encourage departments to put great emphasis on throughput of patients, and students in particular may feel under pressure to work at speed. A balance must be found between caring for the patient who is being examined and not keeping other patients waiting for excessive amounts of time.

Stage 5 – evaluation

Once the initial films have been taken the radiographer will examine them to determine whether the examination is complete or whether further views are required. It is important before leaving the room to check films that the patient's condition is ascertained; certain patients cannot be left alone and they will usually be accompanied to the department. If a patient's condition has deteriorated whilst they are in the department, however, someone must stay with the patient whilst the radiographer examines the images produced. Very often a student will be asked to wait with the patient and this is an opportunity to practise the important skills of patient communication. Talking to the patient in such a situation can help to allay their fears and can do much to make them feel that their needs have been fulfilled whilst in the department. The importance of this skill can never be underestimated. There are certainly occasions where repeat or additional views are required. The radiographer must remember that this can arouse the patient's anxieties as they may be convinced that the additional films are as a result of an abnormality which has been detected. Again, communication is required here to allay the patient's very real fears.

Repeat views may require a return to the adaptation stage of the process to ensure adequate image quality.

Model 2 – circular (holistic)

The alternative model of the process is shown in Fig. 1.2. The model is circular in shape and is described as being more holistic in that it depicts the examination as a whole process rather than the linear model which breaks the examination down into steps or sequences. The linear model has been shown in the discussion above to have overlapping stages; sequencing and assessment may need to occur throughout the examination, for example, and are not necessarily discrete steps in the process. The features of the holistic model are not shown in any critical order, which is intended to underline the fact that in this model the process is seen as being continuous, rather than merely a linear model turned on its side. The inclusion of the terms 'speed' and 'efficiency' here underline the resource pressure felt by the radiographers who originated this version of the model.

Here, patient care and patient communication are shown as integral parts of the process, rather than perhaps being added on to the linear model. This model is analysed in Chapter 14 on work with trauma patients.

Summary

By introducing the concept of a continuum of health, with individuals moving between different points at various stages in their lifespan, this chapter has attempted to place radiography in a broad framework of health care. The key word here for student radiographers is *individuals*. For too long radiography has viewed patients using the biomedical model which is reductionist in character, describing patients in terms of their symptoms. This has unfortunately been particularly true of diagnostic radiography where there has been a widespread tendency to refer to patients as simply 'the chest' or 'the lumbar spine on the trolley'. Two models are presented in this chapter which represent the way groups of radiographers may conceptualize the radiographic process as a whole. Both models are currently being formally tested and developed as part of an ongoing programme of research. The models are presented to the reader as a means of stimulating academic debate within the profession. They will provide the student with an introduction to the place of radiography within the broader context of health care and a framework within which they may develop a holistic view of patients which may improve standards of care in the future.

References

Castle, A. (1988) Concepts of health in diagnostic radiography. *Radiography*, 54 (613), 25–8.

Chesney, D.N. & Chesney, M.O. (1986) *Care of the Patient in Diagnostic Radiography*, (page 1), 6th edn., Blackwell Science Ltd, Oxford.

Culmer, P. (1994) *Trauma Radiography – Modelling the Radiographic Process*, Poster presentation: College of Radiographers' Annual Conference, Harrogate, May 1994.

Dwane, J. (1993) Initial patient contact in diagnostic radiography. *Radiography Today*, 59 (668), 17–18.

Ehrlich, R.A. & McCloskey, E.D. (1989) *Patient Care in Radiography*, 3rd edn. (pages 22–30), C.V. Mosby Co, St Louis.

Makely, S. (1990) Methods for teaching effective patient communication techniques to radiography students. *Radiography Today*, 56 (638), 14–15.

McClellan, M. (1990) The radiographer and the well-woman. *Radiography Today*, 56 (640), 26.

Roper, N., Logan, W.N. & Tierney, A.J. (1980) *The Elements of Nursing*, (pages 22–4), Churchill Livingstone, Edinburgh.

Torres, L.S. (1989) *Basic Medical Techniques and Patient Care for Radiologic Technologists*, (pages 6–11), J.B. Lippincott Co, Philadelphia.

Chapter 2
Aspects of Patient Management

Something of the required approach to the patient has been indicated in the previous chapter, and it will now be considered in further and more practical detail.

Departmental planning and the safety of the patient

The safety of the patient in the X-ray department has been said to be extremely important. If safety is defined as freedom from danger and absence of risk, we have to recognize that safety is something that cannot be obtained for our patients. Patients submitting themselves for X-ray examination are undergoing procedures which have certain inherent risks: these risks are accepted when balanced against the different risks implied in not undertaking the radiological examination. The best we can do for our patients is to minimize and contain the risks which are unavoidable and take out those risks which can be removed. The question to be asked is *not* 'How can we ensure the safety of the patient?' but *is* 'How can we reduce the risks?'

Leaving aside the special risks peculiar to the uses of X-ray equipment, of ionizing radiation and of radiological contrast agents, we find that there are many aspects of departmental planning and organization to be considered if the risks to the patient are comprehensively to be minimized. Below is a list of some of the factors involved and we begin at the initial planning of a new X-ray department.

(1) **Predictable workloads, the size of the department and the possibilities for expansion in the future.** A department which is too small for the work which it must handle is a department with more potential hazards. For example, overcrowding and lack of facilities make infection spread more easily, render high standards of work difficult to achieve and increase frustration, irascibility and carelessness in human beings: the general level of risk rises alarmingly.

(2) **General planning.** Are the traffic flows carefully considered to reduce unnecessary and repetitive travel, prevent intersection of busy routes

for patients and staff and eliminate areas of obstruction? If the general planning is poor, accidents are more likely to happen.

(3) **The available facilities and amenities.** We must take into account here the needs not only of the patients but also of the staff so that they may work well and keep high standards in all aspects of their tasks to produce diagnostic images and to care for patients. The needs of staff and of patients must be in balance.

(4) **Many other safety factors** such as:
   (a) Lighting – good or poor?
   (b) Floor coverings – slippery or not?
   (c) Stairways – steep or not, with handrails or not?
   (d) Any blind corners?
   (e) Good signposting and directional aids – a lost patient may wander into a dangerous situation and have an accident.

(5) **Staffing and the organization of work.** The best designed and equipped department becomes inadequate and hazardous if it is insufficiently staffed and there are not enough people in all grades (from consultant radiologists to cleaners) with the required training to enable them to do the work effectively. Similarly it is damaging if the staff are on the payroll but not there at the time when the work presents itself: efficient departmental organization has its own importance in departmental reduction of risk. (See also Chapter 14 – Major Accident Procedure.)

(6) **The patient's waiting time.** The Patient's Charter has led to the introduction of minimum waiting time standards in many departments. It must be remembered that patients are very anxious when coming for an investigation and this is likely to be exacerbated if waiting times are prolonged. Attention must be given during the planning of any department to the design and facilities in waiting areas. If possible they should be relatively spacious with plenty of chairs provided, and include a separate area for trolleys and patients in wheelchairs. Many departments now also provide play areas for children in a corner of the waiting room, which may be equipped with a range of toys and games.

   The addition of plants, magazines and increasingly even television sets in waiting areas all help to make the waiting period a little easier. It is important that patients are notified of the reason for (and potential length of) any delays. Research has shown that patient anxiety can be reduced by the provision of clear information (Baker, 1992).

(7) **Cleaning the department and keeping it tidy.** These two points hardly need explanation since it is obvious that a department which is dirty or untidy (or both) must present hazards to health and safety. Dirt makes infection spread more easily, and people can fall over filing drawers which have carelessly been left open!

(8) Provision for disabled patients. Departmental planning must take account of all patients who may attend the department, not just those who are able-bodied. An example of lack of thought is seen in hospitals who require their patients to follow coloured lines on the walls to reach other departments. There seems to be an assumption in some places that all blind patients will be accompanied by someone sighted. This is not always the case.

Departmental design must make provision for patients in wheelchairs, including wheelchair access cubicles with wider doors; toilets with sufficient space for wheelchair access, low level toilets and washbasins and the provision of panic button or cords for patients needing urgent assistance.

Initial patient contact

As mentioned in Chapter 1, the room must be prepared in advance with all equipment available which might be required during the examination. It is important psychologically to present the patient with an image of an efficient department. This includes clean and tidy rooms and radiographers who look professional. The first contact with the patient should reinforce this professional image. As Dwane (1993) states: 'The feelings, comfort and kind treatment of the patient may be as significant as the radiograph itself.' Dwane comments on the importance of body posture and a smiling facial expression which gives the patient a feeling of welcome. All patients should be addressed as Mr, Mrs or Miss according to the information given on the card. The temptation to use diminutives must be avoided as they detract from the patient's dignity and individuality (Knowles, 1987).

Once in the X-ray room the patient should be asked to tell you their full name and address as an identity check. It is not sufficient to read the details to a patient and merely ask if they are correct. If there is any query as to the patient's identity the date of birth should also be checked. If the examination is one which has necessitated preparation beforehand the patient should be questioned to ensure that they have complied before commencing (see Chapter 5).

Moving chair and stretcher patients

If the patient is fully mobile getting them onto the X-ray table requires little difficulty after an explanation has been given as to what is required. A step should be provided, or a variable height table brought down to its lowest level, and it is important to safeguard the patient to ensure that they do not bang their head on the tube, for example.

Patients who are not ambulant present special circumstances however. They may reach the department by one of three forms of transport:

(1) Wheelchair,
(2) Trolley,
(3) In the bed which he/she occupies on the ward.

Back problems among radiographers have been the subject of recent research (Darnell, 1992; Eckloff, 1993) and a new EC Directive which came into force on 1 January 1993 supplements the requirements of the Health & Safety at Work Act 1974 and means that manual handling of non-ambulant patients should now be avoided (Corlett *et el.*, 1992). The net effect of this has also been to condemn certain lifting practices (which were previously accepted as normal) as unsafe. The reasons for this are outlined below.

Lifting weights

In lifting a weight, you must consider the following points:

(1) Your centre of gravity, which is located about the level of the second sacral vertebra;
(2) Your base, which is that part of your body which is in contact with the ground and obviously must be the soles of your feet when you are standing;
(3) Your balance, i.e. the fact that if your centre of gravity is over your base you are balanced and will not fall over and that the larger your base the greater the stability, for it is bound to be easier to maintain a centre of gravity over a larger than over a smaller area of base.

When you are standing, you can easily broaden your base simply by putting your feet at some distance apart from each other. As shown in Fig. 2.1 the separation can be achieved in two ways:

(1) By moving the feet apart from each other to either side of the body's mid-line, which is called stride-standing;
(2) By separating the feet so that one is in front of the other, as would be the footprints of someone walking, which (not surprisingly) is called walk-standing.

In both cases it is important that the feet point forwards with their long axes parallel. The choice of stance depends on where you are standing, on what space is available and on the nature of the lifting task.

To preserve your spine when you lift a heavy weight, the important rule is that you must keep your back straight and do not bend it. So you must

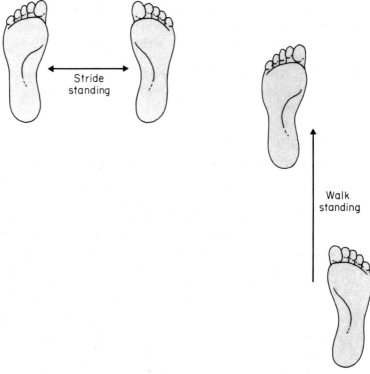

Fig. 2.1 Placement of feet to ensure a wide and stable lifting base.

place yourself as close as you can to whatever you are trying to lift and you must get down to the lift by bending your hips and knees (flexing knee and hip joints) while keeping your spine straight (see Fig. 2.2). You can then lift

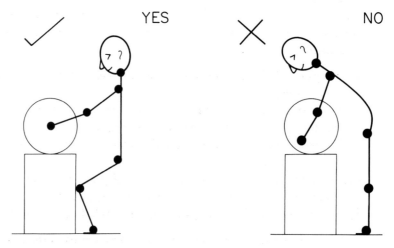

Fig. 2.2 Correct lifting posture for preservation of the spine.

by straightening your legs (extending knee and hip joints) and your spine is spared great stress: thus you can lift a heavy weight much more easily.

So the two basic rules to be remembered are:

(1) Secure your stability by considered placing of your feet;
(2) Lock your spine straight and bend your hips and knees as necessary.

Assessment of patient handling requirements and risk factors

The Manual Handling of Loads Directive requires 'that employers carry out a systematic assessment of the risks of injury arising from manual handling operations and of the action required to reduce those risks to the lowest level reasonably practicable' (HSC, 1992). This is therefore a statutory responsibility. The overall assessment of risk in an imaging department is the responsibility of the superintendent radiographer or imaging services manager. Steps must then be taken as appropriate to reduce the risk to the lowest possible level. These steps will include the purchase of such mechanical aids and manual handling devices as will aid in the reduction of the risks identified. Training must then be provided before any manual handling tasks are undertaken. The use of three typical devices will be described below, but it cannot be stressed too highly that you must receive further practical training before attempting to use any such equipment and that once you have been trained there is a statutory responsibility placed upon you by the Health & Safety at Work Act 1974 and the Manual Handling Regulations to put such training into effect.

Once training has taken place, there is further responsibility placed on individual members of staff to assess a specific lifting task. That individual has to identify the safest way to perform the task and the particular equipment and assistance required to perform it (Corlett *et al.*, 1992). These authors identify a number of factors which must be taken into account in the assessment of the lift:

(1) **Purpose of the lift,** including starting and end points (e.g. trolley to X-ray table),
(2) **Patient data,** including height, weight, ability to co-operate and other constraints such as intravenous drips, splints, etc.,
(3) **Environmental factors,** including furniture, position of X-ray tube and other equipment,
(4) **Selection of transfer/lifting technique,** including mechanical/ manual decision, lifting height involved, posture, etc.
(5) **Equipment and handlers available,** including their skills.

Once all of these factors have been considered in turn, the lift or transfer can be commenced.

The patient in a wheelchair

The patient in a wheelchair will require assistance, in relation to the degree of co-operation they can give. The chair should be brought close to the X-ray table and parallel to it, the patient facing towards the end of the X-ray table at which it is designed to put their feet when they lie down.

In controlling the wheelchair itself there are two points to watch:

(1) That it does not slide away from the patient as they rise,
(2) That the patient is not allowed to stand on the footrest as this will tip the whole chair forwards. On some chairs this can be avoided as the footrest will slide under the seat or will fold away. Other wheelchairs are designed to have stability so that even with someone standing on the foot-rest the chair does not tip.

If the patient is able to stand with some assistance the transfer from chair to table can be effected with the aid of a patient handling sling. The radiographer should place the wheelchair at 90° to the X-ray couch. If the

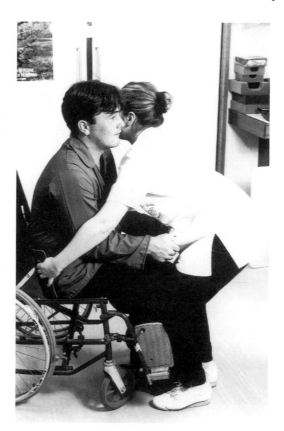

Fig. 2.3 Preparing to transfer with a patient handling sling.

table has a variable-height facility it should be brought down to the same height as that of the wheelchair. The radiographer faces the patient and places their feet in the 'ten-to-two' position to block the patient's feet. The brakes of the chair must be on and if the sides can be removed this will aid the positioning of the lifting sling. Hollis (1991) suggests that the patient hook their thumbs into the radiographer's waist pockets to aid leverage. The radiographer then flexes their hips and knees, so that their knees are placed either side of the patient's knees (again a 'blocking' move). The sling is then placed behind the patient as illustrated in Fig. 2.3. The sling is initially used to transfer the patient in small stages to the front of the seat. The patient is then lifted towards the radiographer (see Fig. 2.4) and transferred through 90° on to the X-ray table. The sling can similarly be used to manoeuvre the patient into the centre of the table.

If the patient is unable to stand, the next safest method of transfer is with the aid of a mechanical hoist. A variety of these is available and radiographers must be trained in the use of the particular model employed in

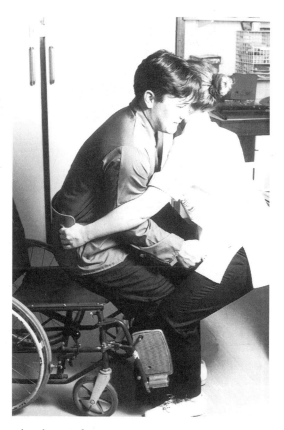

Fig. 2.4 Commencing the transfer.

their departments. The model illustrated in Figs. 2.5 and 2.6 is a mechanized hoist. A canvas is placed under the patient and attached as directed to the hoist mechanism which, when the patient is safely attached, can be raised and swung around over the table and the patient lowered onto the table top.

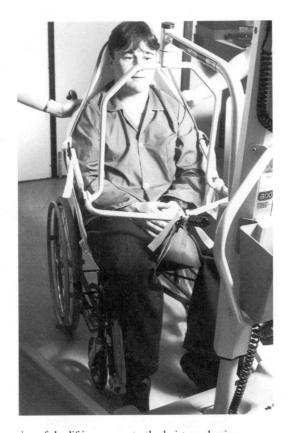

Fig. 2.5 Connection of the lifting canvas to the hoist mechanism.

If a hoist is not available then as a last resort, provided the patient weighs less than 50 kg (8 st), they may be transferred by two radiographers using a shoulder lift (also known as the Australian lift). This is facilitated by the use of a patient handling sling if available. The wheelchair should again be placed at 90° to the table with the brakes on and sides removed if possible. The two radiographers who are to lift should ideally be of similar build; they both stand facing the patient, one on each side. The one on the patient's left puts their left shoulder under the patient's left axilla, and the one on the patient's right side puts their right shoulder under the patient's right axilla (see Fig. 2.7). The radiographers join hands under the patient's buttocks/

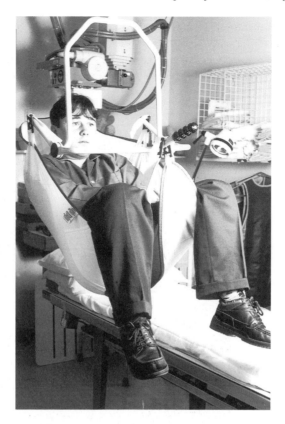

Fig. 2.6 With the hoist raised.

upper thighs or use the lifting sling (Corlett *et al.*, 1992). This lift has been criticized, but the availability of the lifting sling makes it safe because the latter takes the weight of the patient. The radiographers' other hands are clasped behind the patient's back using a double wrist hold as in Fig. 2.8. One of the radiographers must co-ordinate the lift, using clear instructions to the other 'Ready, steady, LIFT'. The radiographers together then lift, step backwards, and, keeping a wide stance and turning together through 90°, transfer the patient onto the X-ray table.

The patient on a stretcher

The *stretcher* patient can be moved on to the X-ray table from the stretcher in a variety of ways, choice depending on the condition of the patient and the general circumstances.

Again the use of devices to facilitate patient transfer must be a priority. Sliding devices provide the easiest means of transferring patients and are

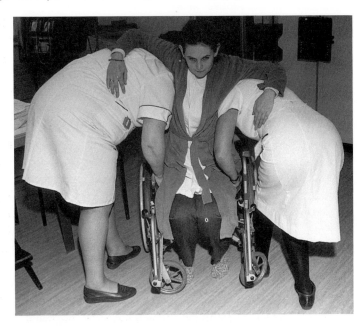

Fig. 2.7 Lifting from a wheelchair a patient unable to help herself. Each radiographer's shoulder is placed in the patient's axilla. The radiographers are placing the lifting sling securely under the patient in preparation for the lift.

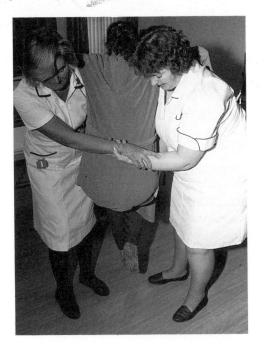

Fig. 2.8 View from behind showing patient supported by the lifting sling. Note the wrist grip used by the two radiographers behind the patient's back.

now being used in many departments. The use of one such device, the 'patslide', is described here. The device is a flat sheet 180 cm (6 ft) long with handholds on each long edge. In order to use such a device the patient must be placed on a canvas or special lifting sheet. Four lifters are required. The trolley is placed alongside the X-ray table and flush with it and the trolley and table brakes must be on. Two lifters are placed on each side of the patient; two at the side of the trolley and two on the far side of the table. The two lifters on the trolley side of the patient grasp the opposite edges of the lifting sheet and gently roll the patient to face them. The two lifters on the far side of the X-ray table then place the 'patslide' in place so that it straddles the trolley and the X-ray table (see Fig. 2.9). The patient is then allowed to lie flat again and the two lifters on the far side of the X-ray table prepare to make the transfer by placing one knee on the X-ray table. In doing so they are able to pull the patient safely towards them, keeping a straight back and with a stable base (see Fig 2.10). The knee on the table allows the lifters to extend their reach further forwards in a safe manner and also evens out any height differences between the two lifters. This is by far the safest method of transferring patients as the movement is a sliding one; there is no actual lifting involved.

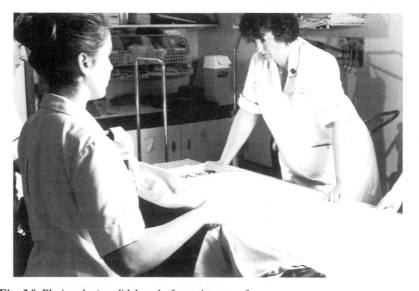

Fig. 2.9 Placing the 'patslide' ready for patient transfer.

It is frequently necessary to turn patients on the X-ray table on to one side for a lateral projection. If the patient is unable to help, it is again important to see that this is done in the proper way, so that both staff and patient are involved in the least expenditure of effort.

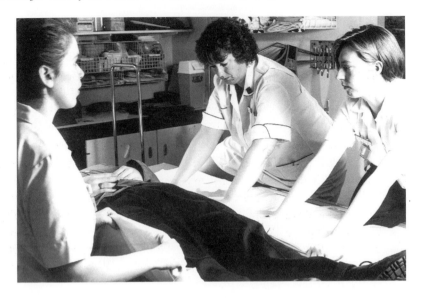

Fig. 2.10 Preparing to move the patient onto the X-ray table.

Since the X-ray table is not very wide it is wise to begin by pulling the patient from the centre of the table nearer to the edge towards which they are *not* going to turn. The patient is less likely then to find that as they turn they roll perilously close to the table edge on the side towards which they are turning.

The turning procedure is begun by alteration in the position of the patient's limbs. If the patient is to be turned on to their *left* side, their left arm is brought away from the body, abducted at the shoulder. The right leg is brought across the trunk, flexed at hip and knee, and the right arm brought forward across the chest. This positioning of the limbs tilts the trunk in the direction of the patient's turn.

The radiographer who will do most of the work of turning the patient (and can in fact act unaided) then goes round the X-ray table to the patient's left side and puts both hands well under the patient, one under the shoulders and one under the pelvis. This is easy to do as the patient's body is already tilted by the weight of the limbs.

It is now possible smoothly and gently to roll the patient on to their left side by the radiographer leaning backwards and pressing with thighs and knees against the X-ray table. Some assistance can be given by another radiographer standing on the other side of the X-ray table, but it will probably not be necessary unless the patient is entirely a dead weight. A patient can be turned from the supine position on to their *right* side in a similar manner with the above procedure reversed as to side.

In moving and turning patients, in picking them up and in putting them down, and in assisting them to move themselves, it is important always to be as smooth and gentle in action as possible. Whenever the X-ray examination is likely to be prolonged in time, it is a kindness to the patient to make the table a softer bed by the use of the thin radiolucent mattresses which are available.

Before beginning any turning movements it is wise to find out whether there is any particular part of the patient which is painful or tender. The patient will wish to guard it from sudden contacts, and it may be necessary to arrange special support for an injured limb, someone being detailed to care for this while the movements are undertaken.

In accident and emergency X-ray departments special casualty trolleys or transport tables are sometimes used. A patient occupying such equipment is seriously injured and should not be moved from it. The design of each system – there are several available – is intended to facilitate radiological investigation with minimum disturbance of the subject (Carter, 1994).

The management of aggression

Any member of hospital staff who comes into direct contact with patients (and with those who accompany or visit patients) should expect sometimes to encounter aggression. Aggressive attitudes hold the possibility of serious hostility and actual physical violence: this potentiality must be recognized and anticipated. The management of aggression is significant in caring for not only those who present the antagonism but also others who may become its victims. It is intended here to leave out the special cases of psychiatric patients and to consider only the circumstances that radiographers might expect in busy general departments, especially those which provide an accident and emergency service.

Causes of aggression

Aggressive attitudes in patients and in those who are with them are caused by multiple factors and do not have single points of origin. Some of the factors are enumerated below.

(1) **The stressful situation.** These people are full of uncertainties, anxieties, shock, pain and fear. Some of them will be better than others in dealing with these strains: for the less able, the tension of their inability to sustain the stress may be transferred to aggression and hostility towards the hospital environment and its staff.

(2) **Frustration.** A definition of frustration is discontentment at inability

to achieve one's desires. People in disagreeable and unfamiliar situations which they themselves cannot improve are likely to feel frustrated.

(3) **Feelings of insecurity.** These are caused by the uncertainties of the situation. What is going to happen? How long will it last? Will it hurt? How soon will things improve? When can we go home? Am I going to have to stay in hospital? How long for? These apprehensions are not allayed if there is little information or explanation available from hospital staff.

(4) **Boredom.** This may be a problem whenever people must spend a period of time with nothing to relieve their forced inactivity. You should not suppose that people cannot be both bored and anxious at the same time: they can. The one state does not necessarily exclude the other and indeed the boredom can exacerbate the anxiety.

(5) **Overcrowding and restricted movement.** The effects on behaviour of crowding and restriction have been scientifically studied both in humans and in animals. It has been recognized, with other things, that aggressive behaviour among monkeys can be produced by over-crowding them in a cage. Too many people in too small a waiting area are in a not dissimilar situation!

(6) **A lowered flashpoint at which self-control is lost.** It can be expected that people who have addictions to drugs or alcohol reach much more quickly the point at which they lose control and their states of mind are even more dangerously explosive if they feel despair towards their addictions. In regard to alcohol of course it does not need a confirmed addiction to lower the level at which self-control of temper is lost: anyone after a few drinks may be readily aggressive.

(7) **Feelings of being ignored or of being casually, insensitively or condescendingly treated.**

If you now read again the seven points enumerated above, thinking of how knowledge of them might be used to reduce aggression, you will realize that much can be done. We cannot immediately alter an individual's ability to stand stress but we can relieve the stress. We cannot entirely remove the sense of insecurity but we can allay it. We can plan to prevent overcrowding and reduce boredom. We can remove the possibility of hurt feelings by control of our own attitudes, our own reactions and our own speech.

Guidelines on aggression

It is not a difficult task to relieve the stress, frustration and feelings of insecurity which those who come to hospital may unpleasantly experience. If you consider the following points you will see that a great deal can be simply done.

(1) Radiographers must preserve a calm, professional, reassuring attitude and must not react to aggressive behaviour by themselves assuming hostility. To maintain your own calm, consciously slow your rate of breathing and breathe more deeply; pitch your voice low and keep emotion out of it; concentrate on noticing and understanding the other person. In some circumstances a radiographer may feel more stressed than the patient. For example, inadequate staffing levels and unpredictable workloads can put the radiographer into a tense state. Doubtless a starting point in the control of aggression in the department is good management so that the staff can do their work with the least stress to themselves. Yet we must remember that whatever our situation *we* are the professionals. Patients have a right to expect that we can control violence not only in others but in ourselves. It is clear that if we cannot achieve the second one, we are crippled as we try to handle the first.

(2) A radiographer's perceptive attitude towards a patient or their companions with an aggressive approach is extremely important. If you can realize that essentially these people are reacting unfavourably not to you as a person but to the stressful circumstances in which they are then you will understand them. This puts you into a position of strength and not into one of weakness and defence. You will be better able to stay calm and in control of yourself and the situation.

(3) Your sympathetic perceptions of the aggressor will be of limited value if you do not also consider carefully the signals which you are sending out for them to perceive in their turn. Remember that these signals are embodied not only in words but also in the tone of your voice and in non-verbal forms of communication. So your speech must be courteous and must avoid the two extremes of overbearing command and complete indifference. You must remember that a stance with your hands on your hips looks antagonistic and that one with your arms folded across your chest implies that you do not want to make contact with whoever is confronting you. If you do not face and directly look at the aggressor you appear evasive and withdrawn.

(4) If the confrontation is becoming seriously hostile you must be even more careful about what you do because you must not convey even the slightest impression that you are about to take violent action yourself. So do not put your hands in your pockets and do try to keep them below waist level. Do not use your hands to make gestures towards the aggressor or to push them further away from you. Do not get closer to the person confronting you than the nearness of the usual conversational distance. We all of us have an instinctive sense of a space around us which is our own

personal territory and when strangers appear to invade it we become uneasy: think how we all feel closed up together in a crowded lift or in a train. On the other hand if you stand too far away you look like someone trying to evade the whole situation and put a barrier to communication with the other person. This may increase the aggressor's frustration and push him nearer to physical violence and in any case it weakens your control of the matter.

(5) Do not appear to dismiss the patient or their companions by tossing your head, shrugging your shoulders, scornfully raising your eyebrows, ignoring any questions, breaking off conversation, laughing and talking with your colleagues in an exclusive way.

(6) Give the patient and their companions a flow of as much information as you can about what you are going to do, what is likely to happen, what they will have to wait for and for how long. You should try to make all this as reassuring and hopeful as you can and explain any difficulties without being too pessimistic about them but you must not deal out evasions and mis-information: for example, saying, 'You'll only have to wait five minutes' when you know that it is likely to be half an hour. Fifteen minutes later the misinformed person may be very agitated and uncertain.

(7) If there is a waiting area in your department it is worth considering what improvements might be made. So assess your waiting area by considering the following questions. Is it large enough to accommodate easily the numbers likely to be in it together? Is it comfortably furnished with good chairs well arranged? Is its scheme of decoration very dreary? Has it facilities such as magazines, toys for children, decorative features such as plants, pictures or a tank of fish to watch? Is there a pay-telephone so that the people can tell those at home or at work what is happening to them? Are there any possibilities for small refreshments such as cups of tea or coffee? Are there visible indications as to where the toilet facilities are? It may be impossible to provide the refreshments or the telephone but clear infor-mation as to where these are to be found is certainly better than ignoring the frustrations that can accumulate in the absence of such facilities. Is it relatively easy for people in the waiting area to have access to staff? Or will they feel that they are remotely closed away with physical barriers between them and the staff so that they cannot get their questions answered? What is the level of noise that has to be tolerated? What might be done to reduce it? What should be done to contain disturbing sounds: for example, children crying and the unmistakable noises of such physical distresses as vomiting and severe pain?

(8) There must be in the department an easily accessible and understood means of summoning effective assistance.

Imminent and actual violence

Throughout the course of an aggressive confrontation the radiographer must observe the other person and assess emotional states, looking for signs of readiness for physical violence. The signs of increasing aggression are:

- Raised voice
- Verbal abuse and other threatening sounds
- Changes of facial colour to be seen in the light-skinned
- Changes in respiration with rate and depth increased
- Restlessness
- Tensing of muscles (visible in face and hands)
- Threatening gestures
- Slight withdrawal if you try to come closer

It is not possible here to lay down firm and never-failing rules for dealing with situations which tend towards, or actually break out into, violence, since such situations and circumstances are all different. However, it is possible to enumerate some points which may be of help.

(1) Your best stance is a balanced one, facing your aggressor with your feet slightly apart, the dominant foot being slightly at the rear and the lesser one being slightly forward with the leg slightly bent. Be careful not to make this stance look too obviously one of preparation for action or you will look threatening yourself.

(2) Your best position is slightly off the intimidator's centre towards their less strong side (if you can identify whether they are right or left handed) slightly out of arm's reach (if you can estimate the length of their arms).

(3) Keep your eyes on a point at the base of the aggressor's neck approximately at the anatomical level of the suprasternal notch. Do not watch the person's eyes for it is more important to get notice of bodily movements and movements of the hands and this the lower level of viewpoint allows you to do. Furthermore it lessens the risk that a fixed eye-contact will be regarded as threatening. You must aim to minimize your own appearance as a threat which may precipitate the person into violence.

(4) In assessing the possibility of damage to people and property, remember that people are the more important.

(5) Try to break away from an attack.

(6) Try to avoid putting others at risk.

(7) If you must physically restrain someone:
    (a) Hold clothing rather than limbs;
    (b) Grasp legs and arms near joints;

(c) Pin the violent person's arms to their body with a bear-hug from the rear;

(d) Restraining weight can be put upon a violent person if they are lain on the floor and others place themselves across the person's body, the most important single area to place the restraining weight being the hips and buttocks;

(e) The degree of force used in restraint must be only as much as is reasonable and it must be applied for no longer than is necessary.

After any episode of severe aggression and violence is over, a full report and record must be made to accord with the rules of procedure which apply to your department. The report must cover the following details:

(1) What happened;
(2) Where and when it happened;
(3) The names and identities of those involved;
(4) The actions taken;
(5) The results of the incident.

References

Baker, D. (1992) Information sheets as a means of reducing patient anxiety during visits to diagnostic imaging departments. *Radiography Today*, 58 (659), 22–4.

Carter, P.H. (1994) *Chesney's Equipment for Student Radiographers*, (p. 154), 4th Edn., Blackwell Science, Oxford.

Corlett, E.T., Lloyd, P.V., Tarling, C., Troup, J.D.G., & Wright, B. *et al.* (1992) *The Guide to the Handling of Patients*, National Back Pain Association, Teddington.

Darnell, C. (1992) The incidence, causes and effects of back pain among diagnostic radiographers. *Radiography Today* 58 (660), 21–3.

Dwane, J. (1993) Initial patient contact in diagnostic radiography. *Radiography Today*, 59 (668), 17–18.

Eckloff, K. (1993) Back problems among diagnostic radiographers. *Radiography Today*, 59 (673), 17–20.

Health & Safety Commission (1992) *Guidance on Manual Handling of Loads in the Health Services*, HMSO.

Hollis, M. (1991) *Safer Lifting for Patient Care*, 3rd Edn., Blackwell Science, Oxford.

Knowles, R. (1987) Who's a pretty girl then? *Nursing Times*, 83 (27), 58–9.

Further reading and relevant legislation

Manual Handling Operations Regulations 1992 (Health & Safety Executive)
Owens, R.G. & Ashcroft J.B. (1985) *Violence: a Guide for the Caring Professions*, Croom Helm Ltd, Kent.

Chapter 3
Drugs in the Imaging Department

A drug may be defined as 'an original simple medicinal substance'. Modern medical practice employs such a full range of materials administered to the patient that this dictionary definition may seem inadequate in its scope. Perhaps then a more acceptable definition of a drug used in medical practice would be 'anything given to a patient to produce an improvement in their condition'. In the X-ray department few substances given to the patient and introduced into the various anatomical and physiological systems are medicinal in the sense that they have healing properties, though they do have attributes adapted to medical use. The range of such substances is limited relative to the wide variety used throughout the hospital.

Defined for the purposes of consideration here as substances administered to the patient, drugs in the X-ray department will be seen to fall into three main groups.

(1) Drugs to be used in preparation of the patient.
(2) Contrast agents for use in X-ray examination of the patient.
(3) Drugs to be used in resuscitation.

The contrast agents from the largest and most extensively used group. In the United Kingdom the usage of drugs is controlled by certain Acts of Parliament and there are regulations which must be followed in keeping drugs in the department.

Medicines and controlled drugs

Acts which affect the present keeping and handling of drugs within the United Kingdom are The Misuse of Drugs Act 1971 and The Medicines Act 1968. From these Acts arise regulations which are concerned with the following, among other matters:

(1) Naming the drugs to which they apply
(2) Storage of the drugs;
(3) Prescriptions for the drugs;
(4) Checks to be made;
(5) Records of stocks and the use made of the drugs.

The Misuse of Drugs Act 1971 affects medicines known as Controlled Drugs (CDs), these being drugs which are liable to misuse; misuse implies that these drugs are habit-forming and are drugs of addiction which people will misuse for the sensations that the drugs give them. This misuse contrasts with their correct use as therapeutic agents, according to doctors' prescriptions. Cocaine, heroin, morphine, pethidine and amphetamine preparations are examples of CDs.

Controlled Drugs are issued only on the written prescription of a medical practitioner, but hospital wards and special departments may keep a stock of some of the preparations. These must be requisitioned by an order in duplicate in a special book signed by an authorized responsible person in charge of the ward or department. The containers of these drugs must indicate that the drug is controlled and they must be kept in a special locked cupboard, of which the key is held on the person in charge of the department responsible for the drugs.

On hospital wards and in radiodiagnostic departments, the substances to which these Acts relate should be held in a designated drug cupboard. This is a cupboard of special design. It incorporates a small inner cupboard for CDs. Both cupboards are lockable; but not with the same key. The drug cupboard – as a whole – and its keys arc in the custody of the appropriate nursing officer or superintendent radiographer concerned. Externally, the cupboard is fitted with a red warning light which illuminates whenever the door is unlocked and serves as a reminder that it must be locked again after use. A lockable drugs refrigerator is also required for drugs needing storage below 8°C (Hopkins, 1992).

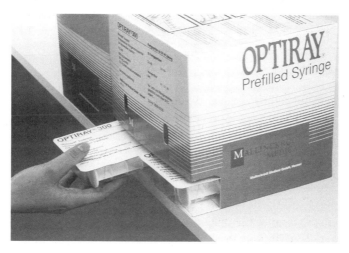

Fig. 3.1 Presentation of iodine-based contrast media in individual sterile packs. (*Reproduced by courtesy of Mallinckrodt Medical (UK) Ltd.*)

Many of the drugs needed in an X-ray department are prepared by the manufacturers in glass bottles which hold more than one dose, the end being closed by a rubber diaphragm which is usually covered with a screw top. Such a bottle should be held by its sides so that the hands do not contaminate the rubber top. The contents are withdrawn by piercing the rubber diaphragm with a needle through which the drug is drawn into a syringe. Contrast agents may also now be presented in the form of pre-filled syringes presented in individual sterile packs.

Units of measurement

The metric system

In the metric system mass is measured in kilograms, grammes, and milligrams. In writing, g is the symbol for a gramme, with kg, and mg for the multiple or fraction of it. Volume is measured in terms of the litre (l), which is the volume of one kilogram of water at 4°C. A fraction of the litre is the millilitre (ml) which is the volume of one gramme of water at the same temperature.

SI units

In the SI system the base unit of length is the metre (symbol m), the base unit of mass is the kilogram (symbol kg) and the unit of volume derived from the base unit of length is the cubic metre (symbol m^3). It is possibly worth noting as an aid to clear and correct expression that these symbols are not followed by full stops and that they do not change in the plural; for example, you correctly write 1 m and 2 m (or whatever quantities you are expressing). The symbols are capital letters only when the unit is called after a proper name: for example, the SI unit of force is the newton and its symbol is N.

The alert reader may notice that the unit of mass is referred to but not the unit of weight. The fact is that the word weight is ambiguous in common usage. Sometimes it means mass and sometimes mechanical force. It has been strictly defined as a quantity of the same nature as a force, the standard weight of a body being the product of its mass and the standard acceleration due to gravity.

SI units have decimal multiples and submultiples which are indicated by prefixes. For example, the prefix *kilo* (symbol k) indicates multiplication by one thousand (it is to be said at this point that the kilogram is the only base unit which has a prefix). The prefix *mega* denotes multiplication by one million, the symbol for this prefix being M. Common submultiples are division by one hundred indicated with the prefix *centi* (c), by one thousand indicated with *milli* (m) and by one million indicated with the prefix *micro* (μ).

Certain units in very wide application are not part of the SI system but are retained for use with it simply because they are so often employed. One of these is the litre as a unit of volume.

Among the SI units is one for amount of substance, used to specify amounts of chemical elements or compounds. This unit is based on the number of atoms in a particular quantity (0.012 kilogram) of a particular isotope of carbon (carbon 12) and it is called the mole (symbol mol). In hospital practice students may encounter its use, for example, to express amounts of inorganic or nitrogenous substances present in a blood sample. Thus in blood plasma the mean value for potassium is 4.30 millimoles per litre (mmol/1) and for urea 4.49 millimoles per litre.

Temperature

In the SI system thermodynamic temperature is expressed in kelvin (symbol K) and Celsius temperature is also used. Celsius temperature is defined by an equation which relates it to kelvins and it is expressed in degrees (Celsius (°C). The kelvin is the unit of absolute temperature and degrees Celsius equate with the Centigrade scale.

In hospital practice body temperature may be expressed in degrees Celsius. The average normal body temperature is 36.8° Celsius and this is comparable with 36.8° Centigrade.

Percentage solutions

The term 'per cent' denotes the strength of a solution. If the solute is a solid it will be measured by weight, the liquid solvent being measured by volume. The strength of the solution will then be given by the expression 'per cent w/v', meaning weight in volume. If the solute and the solvent are both liquids they are measured by volume, and the strength is then given by the expression 'per cent v/v', meaning volume in volume.

Drugs used in preparation of the patient

In the X-ray department drugs may be kept to be used in preparing the patient for X-ray examinations. The range of these is not wide. Certain X-ray examinations (for example, angiography) are very unlikely to be undertaken on outpatients, and if the patient is in hospital the responsibility for preparation will rest with the ward. Drugs from the ward stock will be used in accordance with the recommendations of the X-ray department. However, there are some examinations for which some premedication is required which may well be done on outpatients (e.g. hysterosalpingo-graphy), and it may be useful to keep in the X-ray department a small stock of the necessary drugs. Certain X-ray examinations require the use of a local anaesthetic and this also is something that might be kept in the department.

It can be said that drugs used in preparation are likely to fall within the following general groupings.

(1) Aperients and suppositories;
(2) Sedative drugs such as diazepam (Valium);
(3) Preparations for local anaesthesia such as lignocaine;
(4) Analgesics such as aspirin and paracetamol compounds.

In a radiodiagnostic department only a small quantity of such and other drugs is likely to be kept, but even so their storage and segregation are not exempt from statutory regulation and should follow approved pharmaceutical practice.

A student interested enough to visit a hospital pharmacy may learn something about four classifications which affect the availability of drugs. These are:

(1) General sales list (GSL);
(2) Pharmacy medicines (P);
(3) Prescription only medicines (POM);
(4) Controlled drugs (CD).

We need not study the full implications of these groups (essential knowledge for a pharmacist), but no doubt it is clear to the reader that each classification increasingly restricts the handling and dispensing of the drugs listed within it.

GSL medicines – in certain small quantities only – can be sold freely anywhere, for instance from the shelves of supermarkets. P medicines can be obtained only from a pharmacy; in practice this is often the pharmaceutical section of a chemist's shop. Drugs in the POM list can be obtained only through a doctor's or dentist's prescription; whilst the prescription for a CD medicine must be in the handwriting of the prescriber and its quantities – like those of a cheque – stated in both numerals and words.

The general sales list intrinsically is of scant professional concern to radiographers; and the P list is hardly different in this respect. The statutory information to be printed on the packings of drugs includes a statement of the listing of each. Student radiographers who care to examine the preparations in use in their X-ray departments – and they should take any opportunity to do so – are likely to find that the majority are POM medicines. For example, the tranquillizer diazepam is on the POM list; as also are radiological contrast agents for intravascular administration, and the corticosteroids and antihistamines used to control allergic reactions.

The storage of drugs

In the X-ray department, POM drugs needed during the preparation or treatment of patients are stored under lock and key. Usually this is in the type of cupboard which is specified for the storage of controlled drugs and of which the key will be held by a responsible member of staff, such as a superintendent or senior radiographer, a staff nurse or nursing sister (see this chapter, Medicines and Controlled Drugs). Whilst there is no legal requirement to keep POM drugs under this strict control, the practice is followed in most hospital trusts and similar locations.

The same degree of control hardly needs to be exercised in respect of such drugs as laxatives (which may be P listed); but there should be an invariable rule that preparations suitable only for external application – for instance, antiseptics and disinfectants – are not kept in any cupboard which also contains a medicine. Segregation merely to another shelf is insufficient and hazardous, inviting a possibly deadly error.

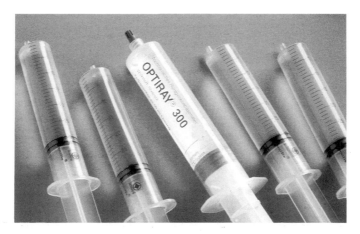

Fig. 3.2 Identification on syringes helps to eliminate error. *(Reproduced by courtesy of Mallinckrodt Medical (UK) Ltd.)*

Regulations for the safe keeping of drugs may have to be relaxed in particular circumstances. These circumstances arise in the X-ray department in providing drugs which may be used in the resuscitation of a patient suffering an adverse reaction to the administration of a radiological contrast agent. In this situation a needed drug which is under lock and key in a cupboard may not come to hand sufficiently quickly to help the patient.

The dilemma to be resolved – by local agreements between the consultant radiologist, the superintendent radiographer and the chief pharmacist – is to decide where the greater risk lies: in the open availability of small quantities of them *not* being readily accessible? Some degree of compromise is possible and to this end the following points should be considered in equipping resuscitation trolleys/emergency drug trays.

(1) The trolley should not be kept in any place where many people – especially members of the public – would normally pass, for example in a corridor. It should stand, if possible, in an X-ray room where it is likely to be used.
(2) The provision of a loose cover (of linen or plastic material) over the trolley serves the double purpose of protecting the equipment from dust and preventing its contents from being directly visible. Such a cover can be made to drape over the whole trolley to be readily lifted by means of looped handles on the top.
(3) Emergency drug trays may be located in other X-ray rooms such as that used for intravenous urography. These are presented as plastic trays containing an agreed range of drugs for emergency resuscitation, covered with clear film. The trays are marked with an expiry date. When the tray is opened *or* when the expiry date is due (whichever is the sooner) the tray is returned to pharmacy for checking, replenishing and resealing.

Contrast agents used in imaging examinations

The term *contrast agents* denotes substances which can be used to show organs or parts of the body in radiographic contrast to their surrounding tissues. The contrast material achieves this result in one of two ways. Either it is of low atomic number and causes the part in which it is placed to be *more* readily penetrated by X-rays than is the surrounding tissue; this is called a negative contrast agent. Or it is of high atomic number and causes the part in which it is placed to be *less* readily penetrated by X-rays than is the surrounding tissue; this is called a positive contrast agent and it may also be described as an opaque medium.

It should be noted that the expression *an opaque medium* is a correct singular form. The plural is *some opaque media*. The words *contrast medium* and *contrast media* are often encountered in place of *contrast agent* and *contrast agents* and this is correct usage. Unfortunately the tiresome error of *contrast media* used as a *singular* is extremely widespread.

Negative contrast materials

The only negative contrast materials are gases such as air or oxygen or carbon dioxide. Air-filled parts are shown in the radiographic image of an ordinary X-ray film as black areas because the gas is letting through more X-radiation to blacken the film, and on the fluorescent screen as light areas because more X-radiation is being transmitted through the gas to make the screen fluoresce.

For diagnostic purposes air or oxygen or carbon dioxide may be put into tracts and cavities in various systems of the body. Some examples of organs suitable for the injection of a gas are the colon and the joint spaces of the knee.

A natural demonstration of the effectiveness of gas as a negative contrast agent can be found in films of the abdomen taken with the patient erect. The normal 'gas bubble' present in the stomach is then seen readily, and it can be noted that part of the left side of the diaphragm is delineated by reason of its situation between the air-filled lungs above and the gas contained in the stomach immediately below. Air or carbon dioxide are now commonly used to provide double contrast in barium examinations.

Positive contrast materials

Positive contrast agents are all substances of high atomic number which absorb X-radiation. Therefore in the radiographic image of the X-ray film they make structures in which they are present appear more radiopaque in contrast to the surrounding tissue because less radiation is reaching the film to blacken it. Correspondingly they appear dark on the fluorescent screen because less X-radiation is reaching the screen to make it fluoresce.

These contrast materials are used in a variety of ways depending on the material and the part of the body which it is desired to examine. They can be introduced into tracts and cavities, and some of them can be allowed to pass into certain physiological systems so that the function of the organs concerned (for example the kidneys and gall bladder) can be examined radiographically.

Elements of high atomic number which are used to make these pre-parations are (1) barium and (2) iodine.

Barium preparations

Barium is employed as a radiographic contrast agent in the form of one of its salts – barium sulphate. It is used almost solely for examination of all parts of the alimentary tract (the pharynx and oesophagus, the stomach, the small bowel, the colon).

Barium sulphate is chosen for the following reasons.

(1) It has a high atomic number.
(2) It is insoluble and stable, and will pass through the intestinal tract without dissolving or changing to form substances poisonous to the

patient. Salts of barium other than the sulphate are highly poisonous.
(3) It causes little upset to the intestinal tract even in large doses, although it may aggravate a constipated condition.
(4) It has the virtue of being relatively cheap.

Barium sulphate is supplied commercially as a powder or as a ready diluted suspension; in nature this is white but a pink colorant may be present to enhance the eye-appeal of the drink which a patient receives. Any colorant is unnecessary, of course, in the case of a barium sulphate mixture to be given as an enema.

Under various proprietary names, several presentations are available for oral administration and are similar to each other in broad respects. A capped plastic cannister (of about 500 ml capacity) may contain 200–300 g of barium sulphate powder, to which the user adds some 60–80 ml of water. He obtains, thus, a fine suspension of barium sulphate in water at a stated weight/volume ratio. Depending on the purpose for which the suspension is intended, these ratios vary: a high density barium formulation may be used at 200% w/v or 250 w/v. One well known preparation is already in liquid form in a sealed can and has a w/v ratio of 100%. Certain formulations have different additives to aid coating or prevent flocculation, for example.

In the case of a barium formulation prepared for administration as an enema, the container more suitably is a plastic bag, having within it 400–600 g of barium sulphate powder. The user may add to this up to 2000 ml of water and will obtain w/v ratios in the range 20% to 65%. For a double contrast study, a small quantity of water (for instance 500 ml) and consequently higher w/v ratios are appropriate.

Care of barium preparations
With regard to keeping and using barium sulphate preparations in the department, there are some points which should be borne in mind. These may seem so obvious that they take on the appearance of being insignificant, but errors arising from lack of attention to them are potentially disastrous in result. There are on record cases of barium examinations which have been lethal to the patient because of a 'simple' mistake.

Storage conditions are not unduly restrictive. The area should be dry, reasonably cool atmospherically, and socially clean. Preferably the vicinity includes an adequate extent of working space and access to a mains water tap.

The preparations used must be kept in clearly labelled containers, and the radiographer must check the container to make sure that the right preparation is being used. There is not likely to be any difficulty here in the case of the proprietary preparations, for these are of course supplied in containers clearly and durably labelled.

Anyone who prepares a contrast agent in a badly lighted area takes a needless risk. It may seem tiresomely punctilious to find danger in inadequate lighting when custom makes a procedure familiar and practice persuades us that nothing can go wrong. Yet some people have learned from irrevocable experience that had they been able to *see* fully the materials they were using, disaster would not have occurred.

Iodine preparations

Preparations in which molecules of iodine are the opaque agent form a very large group of contrast materials used in many different X-ray examinations.

An important requirement of all these preparations is that they must be stable compounds which do not break down after they have been given to the patient, with possibly dangerous effects.

It is to be noticed that the administration of a contrast agent which contains iodine will prevent the thyroid gland from taking up iodine for a period which may be as long as 10 weeks: this may affect the results of testing using iodine radioisotopes. A patient submitted to both forms of investigation should not have the X-ray examination *before* the organ scan.

Organic iodine compounds have a complex molecular structure, and as a result they tend to have full names which are lengthy and meaningless to those not learned in organic chemistry. In most cases they are called by a shortened name or by trade names under which these various preparations are sold.

Despite their complexity, the molecules of these compounds may be simply considered as having two consistent features: (1) the iodine which provides the radiopaque elements and makes the substance a contrast agent for radiography, and (2) the chemical remainder which holds the iodine in stable combination and determines the chemical, physical, and physiological properties of the compound. In absorption of these agents iodine is excreted by the kidneys, but the carrier factor may remain and form residues which are potentially harmful. This eventuality is one of many which require consideration in the manufacture of new contrast agents.

Increase in the iodine content of each molecule increases the efficacy of the compound in providing contrast which indeed is its only purpose: the more iodine contained in any volume of a solution, the more strongly radiopaque is that solution. Products which are now available generally have 3 or 6 atoms of iodine per molecule.

The organic iodine compounds can be considered from the point of view of the X-ray examinations for which they are used. These fall into three main groups. These groups are:

(1) Organic iodine compounds for intravascular administration;
(2) Organic iodine compounds for oral cholecystography;

(3) Other organic iodine compounds which are *not* for intravascular injection, and are used for contrast examinations which are not included in the previous two groups.

(1) Organic iodine compounds for intravascular administration. There is a numerous group of tri-iodinated organic iodine compounds which may be injected intravascularly; some are suitable also for administration by lumbar puncture during myelography (radiculography). Their various characteristics have been studied at length in clinical trials and the safety and usefulness of each substance deeply debated. Choices between contrast agents are made by radiologists rather than radiographers because of the clinical considerations involved; nevertheless some knowledge of the behaviour of these iodinated compounds is important to anyone who needs to understand their imaging applications.

Many intravascular contrast agents in current use are solutions of the sodium salts or meglumine salts – or a combination of both – of iodinated derivatives of benzoic acid. (Diatrezoic, iothalamic, and metrizoic acids are examples.) These are strong acids and when their soluble salts are put in solution each molecule dissociates, to a sodium or meglumine cation (a positive ion) and an iodinated anion (a negative ion). The importance of these ions in radiodiagnostic practice is that the occurrence of certain adverse reactions to such contrast agents has been ascribed to their presence, particularly to chemotoxic effects from the cations. In this connection, sodium has been shown to have greater toxicity than meglumine, though neither ion is biologically inert.

Apart from possible toxicity of the injected chemical, these ionized solutions have a high osmolality which is extremely damaging potentially to human tissue. These solutions may be referred to generically as high osmolar contrast media (HOCM) (Chapman & Nakielny, 1993). Osmolality refers to the movement of molecules across a membrane between a weak solution and a concentrated one, to which the membrane is impermeable. During angiography, a bolus of a highly concentrated contrast agent temporarily replaces blood flowing through a vessel or group of vessels. The introduction of such a hypertonic solution results in a great shift of intracellular water through cellular membranes; nature attempts to re-establish osmolar equilibrium, and a number of undesirable side effects have been studied in detail and are ascribed to this fluid transference. For instance, pain during anteriography – because blood flow increases locally – is one of these effects; and certain rises in pulmonary arterial pressure which have been noticed are thought to occur because of changes in red blood cells. (It is here obvious that the structures most challenged during arteriography are blood cells and the endothelium of blood vessels.)

From our brief discussion of these problems it can hardly surprise the reader to know that much attention has been given to the synthesis of low osmolar and non-ionic contrast agents; and student radiographers may have heard these terms applied to some contrast agents in use in their training departments. It is to be remarked that the two descriptions do not mean the same thing, as we hope our previous paragraphs have shown. To emphasize this point, a widely available, low osmolar contrast medium (LOCM) contains meglumine and sodium salts of ioxaglic acid and dissociates (ionizes) in solution; but its osmolality is rather less than some non-ionic contrast agents which have been developed and have achieved great reduction in osmolality.

The non-ionic compounds are amide derivatives of other tri-iodinated substituted benzoic acids. The first to enter clinical practice was metriza-mide. Metrizamide, when dissolved in water, does not dissociate and each dissolved molecule contains three atoms of iodine. The aqueous solution is unstable on autoclaving, however, and must be prepared immediately before the examination for which it is to be used. Metrizamide has been extensively employed for myelography (radiculography).

Iohexol, ioversol and iopamidol are more recently developed non-ionic media, of a similar ratio (number of iodine atoms compared with osmotically active particles). They are stable in solution and have wide applications, being suitable for intravascular and subarachnoid injection.

Chemical and osmolar attributes aside, the viscosity of a solution for injection may be physically significant. A viscous solution is difficult for an operator to administer, particularly in the relatively large quantities asso-ciated with intravenous urography and angiography. Among those com-pounds which we have here considered, the sodium salts demonstrably have the lowest viscosity in solution, whilst solutions of iopamidol and iohexol more nearly compare with the viscosity of corresponding solutions of meglumine salts.

To the readers of this book, even the shortened names of the contrast agents described are not closely familiar; much more readily recognizable are the trade names under which different companies offer these medicines. For example, Merck's 'Niopam' is iopamidol; Nyegaard's 'Omnipaque' is iohexol; and May & Baker's 'Hexabrix' is meglumine and sodium ioxaglate. In many instances a number may be combined with the trade name and indicate what we may describe loosely as the 'strength' or contrast-produc-ing capability of the solution. More precisely, the number refers to the quantity of iodine present in 1 millimetre of the solution: 'Hexabrix 320' contains 320 mg combined iodine per millilitre; 'Niopam 300' has 300 mg iodine/ml; 'Omnipaque 350 has 350 mg iodine/ml; and in 'Conray 280' – meglumine iothalamate injection – the numerals have a similar significance.

Students, looking carefully at the different iodinated contrast agents in use in their departments, should be able to recognize their iodine contents per millilitre, and to appreciate how the concentration of the drug may affect its clinical applications. To give but one example, in the case of 'Niopam', the '370' presentation is appropriate for coronary arteriography; and the '200' presentation for contrast enhancement during brain scanning by computed tomography. Such information is more significant practically to radiographers than a specific familiarity with chemical structures.

(2) Organic iodine compounds for oral cholecystography. X-ray examinations of the gall bladder usually involve oral administration of an organic iodine compound and depend upon a *functioning gall bladder* to become filled with the medium. The opaque material reaches the liver via the portal circulation, and is eventually concentrated by the gall bladder. The depth of contrast obtained, that is the degree of opacity of the organ as it appears on the radiograph, depends on the function of the gall bladder mucosa.

Many orally administered contrast agents for cholecystography are available and it is proposed to mention here only a few as examples.

'Biloptin' is a compound of which the approved chemical name is sodium ipodate. It is offered in capsular form: each capsule contains 0.307 g iodine and the normal adult dose is six capsules, comparable to the tablet pre-parations. 'Solu–Biloptin' is calcium ipodate. It appears as a powder in a sachet, each sachet containing 1.85 g iodine. The patient is instructed to put the contents of the sachet in an empty tumbler and stir in a small amount of water or diluted fruit squash before taking.

Children are rarely candidates for cholecystography, but when this is the case tablets are contraindicated and Solu–Biloptin is used.

Because of its fast absorption, Solu–Biloptin is suitable for rapid chole-cystography on unprepared patients: a double dose may be given and films exposed after two and a half to three hours.

'Telepaque' is iopanoic acid and contains 66.68% of organically bound iodine. The presentation is in tablet form, the normal adult dose being 3 g (six tablets); this may safely be doubled if necessary.

(3) Other organic iodine compounds. There is a group of organic iodine compounds which cannot be injected intravascularly. They are used for examinations in which the method of application is the direct filling of a space or potential space, introduction of the material being made either through a natural body orifice or by means of a hollow needle or tube put into the space concerned. The regions for which these organic iodine compounds and these methods are used include principally the following: the spinal canal, the urethra, the uterus, the bile ducts post-operatively through a tube which has been left *in situ*, the ducts of the salivary glands, and the tracts of abnormal sinuses and fistulae.

'Gastrografin' is a contrast agent for special use; in this case the correct application is the alimentary tract, as we might infer from the name. It is a combination of sodium diatrizoate and meglumine diatrizoate in an aqueous solution, with which – since it is to be taken by mouth – a flavouring agent (anise) and a wetting agent (Tween 80) are incorporated. These of course make Gastrografin unsuitable for intra-arterial or intravenous injection, but otherwise it is one of the ionic group of intravascular contrast agents which are described in (1) above.

Because it is a hypertonic solution, the administration of Gastrografin is attended by certain risks for some patients. For instance, someone who has suffered a period of vomiting and diarrhoea is likely to be dehydrated. The introduction then of a hypertonic solution to their gut must worsen their physiological imbalance, as the concentrated solution draws fluid through the bowel wall from other tissue. Gastrografin is also unsuitable for post-operative administration following surgery of the upper gastrointestinal tract: it may be aspirated into the lungs, with severely toxic – even lethal – effects.

The particular advantage of Gastrografin refers to cases of suspected or threatening perforation. Barium sulphate is insoluble and if it enters the peritoneal cavity through a gastric or intestinal leak can be difficult to remove. In the same circumstance, sodium/meglumine diatrizoate is eliminated through the kidneys. Presented as suspensions of an insoluble power, barium sulphate has a clogging effect in the large bowel when ingested, which may aggravate a partial obstruction. For these patients, too, Gastrografin may be of special value.

Because of its high osmotic pressure, Gastrografin should not be given to young children or infants, unless it is diluted with an equal or twice its volume of water, and measures are taken to correct the patient's electrolyte and water balance.

Gastrografin may be used in various dosages, depending on the type of patient, on whether the procedure is a 'meal' or an 'enema', and on whether the Gastrografin is employed by itself or in combination with a suspension of barium sulphate.

Student radiographers are not expected to possess any detailed chemical knowledge of the many organic iodine compounds used in radiology. In this section we have mentioned a number which are appropriate only to mechanical introduction into a body cavity. It is this characteristic which is of serious significance to the radiographer, who – although not directly their user – is often the person preparing the instruments and materials for a particular procedure. The responsibility for administering a contrast agent to a patient is a medical one but this does not alter the desirability of radiographers understanding the nature of these drugs and the dangers of any indiscriminate application.

At the beginning of this section we listed a number of bodily regions for the examination of which this group of organic iodine compounds is suitable. It is possible to employ for certain of these procedures (for example, hysterosalpingography) some of the compounds designated for urography and angiography earlier in this chapter (see (1) Organic Iodine Compounds for Intravascular Administration). However, it is *not* possible to employ for intravenous or intra-arterial injection any of the compounds described here for intra-cavitary introduction.

Contrast agents for magnetic resonance imaging

Contrast agents are now being developed for magnetic resonance imaging which produce changes in relaxation times for protons in different tissues. These produce differential signal enhancement (Chapman & Nakielny 1993, p38). The two agents commercially available at the time of writing are manufactured from paramagnetic substances. The first was called Gadolinium. The chemical name of the agent is *dimeglumine gadopentate ('magnevist')*. Its main advantages are the improved delineation of demyelinating diseases and tumour margins, particularly in the central nervous system. The latest of these contrast agents uses crystals of iron ferrite (*'Abdoscan'*) and can be used to label the bowel during abdominal scanning, facilitating organ delineation and visualization of pathology.

The use of contrast agents

When contrast agents are used in the X-ray department, there are certain points which have to be considered. First of all, the chance of reactions occurring as a result of their being given to the patient. This is particularly important in regard to the iodine compounds intravenously injected. Sensitivity to iodine is not uncommon, and the intravenous injection gives a rapid and systemic dispersal through the blood stream.

The reactions which occur may be mild, such as sensations of warmth, nausea, and faintness, but they can be severe resulting in a shock-like state, and they can be lethal. Methods of dealing with these reactions are discussed in another part of this book (see Chapters 7 and 17).

In preparing to give *any* contrast medium to the patient the radiographer must first make sure that it is the right patient, checking the patient's name against the request form and the examination required. In certain cases the opaque medium will in fact be given to the patient by a doctor (for example, as an intravenous injection), but this does not absolve the radiographer from responsibility. The patient's name must be checked, the opaque agent must be checked when it is selected, when it is given to the patient, and again when the container is returned to wherever it is kept or the empty ampoule discarded. In the case of an intravenous injection the radiographer must see that the doctor also checks the substance before it is given.

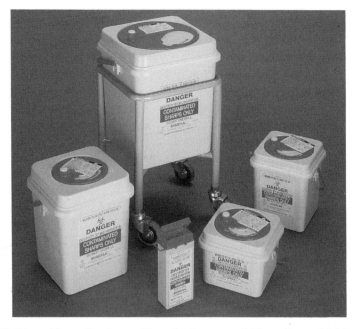

Fig. 3.3 Disposal boxes for sharps. *(Reproduced courtesy of Clinton Patey of DRG Medical Packaging Supplies.)*

Anything given to the patient should never be kept in or issued from an unlabelled container.

Drugs used in resuscitation

It has been indicated that reactions to contrast agents are possible, particularly when they are injected into the bloodstream. Examinations of this type are being carried out by X-ray departments upon increasing numbers of patients. This must raise the risk of 'reaction incidents', and the X-ray department must prepare itself to meet these emergencies.

The time factor is important since for a severe reaction treatment must be instituted *at once*. It is therefore sound practice, indeed essential practice, to have in the X-ray room an emergency supply of various drugs and instruments. These are held ready on a preprepared trolley but the drugs at least should be enclosed in a box which is sealed, but of which the seals may be easily broken.

Chapters 7 and 17 in this book deal in more detail with the treatment of reactions to contrast agents but it can be said that the drugs in an emergency box are likely to include the following.

(1) Adrenaline (1 in 1000) to raise blood pressure and increase cardiac output.
(2) Analeptic drugs for injection. These are drugs which stimulate and restore. One example is aminophylline, which stimulates the muscular tissue of the heart.
(3) Drugs which decrease cardiac excitability, such as lignocaine (2%).
(4) Drugs which reduce allergic reactions in the body. Examples are the corticosteroids and the antihistamines.
(5) An intravenous anaesthetic.
(6) Sterile distilled water for injection (Chapman & Nakielny, 1993, pp 398–402).

If a patient collapses to the extent that his heart stops beating (cardiac arrest) and he stops breathing (respiratory arrest), clearly the first things that must be done for him are to restore the pumping action of the heart and put air into his lungs by mechanical means (see Chapter 17). Once the actions have been established, the medical team will proceed with a therapeutic plan and are likely to give the patient four substances. These are used (1) because the chemistry of the body has been disturbed by what is happening to the patient (his blood, for example, will be somewhat acid instead of being very slightly alkaline as it normally is); (2) because the heart muscle has lost its normal degree of tension and vigour (tone); and (3) because the heart may not resume its normal rhythmic contractions but be in a state of abnormal twitching (fibrillation).

These conditions must be corrected and the substances used are:

(1) Sodium bicarbonate to correct the metabolic acidosis;
(2) Adrenaline to restore the heart tone;
(3) A calcium salt such as calcium chloride which also restores the heart tone and has an enhanced effect when used in conjunction with adrenaline;
(4) Lignocaine, which is a local anaesthetic but in this instance is used for its specific properties affecting the heart muscle. It damps down the irritability of the heart muscle and assists in combating fibrallation.

The above observations are intended only for the general guidance of the student reader. Radiographers do not carry medical responsibility and do not make decisions involving the supply and use of drugs to be employed in a clinical emergency; nor can any particular selection of drugs be regarded as the only correct one in such a situation. Students who enquire about the provisions in their own hospital may find a much lengthier list of substances than the one given here, or may find confusingly different names and presentations. The choice will be influenced by the consultant cardiologist's own opinion of what is appropriate and perhaps also by the geographical situation of the X-ray department: whether it is very distant from effective clinical support or is close to a ward unit. Students who do not understand the contents of the box or trolley kept in the department where they work are well advised to make their own enquiry about it.

Labelling and issuing

It may be emphasized in conclusion that the labelling of all containers is most important. Labels must be placed on the body of the container and not upon the lid. They must be clear, they must not be altered, and if damaged they must be renewed. They should be renewed by returning the container to the hospital pharmacy where the labels will be properly replaced. It must be recognized that once any agents have been separated from their labelled containers opportunity has been made for an element of doubt as to their nature, and contents therefore must not be removed from their containers except for immediate use.

Many of the substances used in the imaging department become very familiar to staff and they are given to many patients each week with no problems at all. However, it is important to be vigilant during such procedures as mistakes can have very serious consequences.

References

Chapman, S. & Nakielny, R. (1993) *A Guide to Radiological Procedures*, (pages 20–42 and 395–402), 3rd Edn., Baillière Tindall, London.

Hopkins, S.J. (1992) *Drugs and Pharmacology for Nurses*, 11th Edn., Churchill Livingstone, Edinburgh.

Further reading

Carr, D.H. (1988) *Contrast Media*, Churchill Livingstone, Edinburgh.

Chapter 4
Sterilization and Sterile Techniques

To sterilize anything for surgical purposes is to make it free from all living organisms. Among these living organisms will be included disease-producing bacteria. Surgical procedures in hospital carry risk of infection and sepsis for the patient, and even when the surgery seems of very minor character (for example, puncturing a vein with a needle to give an intravenous injection) the risk of injection, of bacteria entering the body and growing and multiplying in the tissues, is none the less there.

Patients are susceptible to infection. They are not in a state of full health, and are thus in a weakened condition and less able to combat bacterial invasion. The principle of asepsis in surgery – that is, of applying to surgery techniques which totally exclude the presence of disease-producing organisms – was introduced by Lister, and the low survival rate from surgery in earlier times consequently improved dramatically.

Methods of preventing infection are based upon the fact that bacteria cannot effectively travel by themselves. The ways in which infection can be spread are therefore ways by which bacteria are carried. Bacteria can be conveyed from one person to another and from one place to another in the following ways.

(1) By direct contact. For example, a surgeon who operates with bacteria present on his clothes or hands may transfer these organisms directly to his instruments, and thus to the patient via the operation wound. It is to prevent this type of transfer of bacteria that surgeons not only use instruments and dressings which have been made free from living organisms by sterilization, but also wear sterile gowns over their theatre clothes and sterile gloves on their hands. Anyone assisting a surgeon and handling instruments he will use must take the same precautions.

(2) By aerial carriage. Probably the most important way in which bacteria can be aerially conveyed is by droplet infection. This term refers to direct infection by droplet from the nose and mouth. Certain diseases can be conveyed by those who give no evidence of having the disease and yet have the organisms present in their bodies; these people are called *carriers*. Diphtheria is an example of a disease which can be spread by droplet infection from carriers. In order to prevent spread of bacteria by droplet infection, hospital staff working with sterile equipment in conditions of surgical asepsis wear a mask which covers both mouth and nose and is designed to act as a barrier.

(3) Food and water carriage. Food and water are often vehicles for the transport of bacteria. Typhoid fever may be considered as a typical example of the way in which infection may be so conveyed from one place to another. Typhoid fever is a disease of the intestine, and the organisms are present in the faeces and sometimes the urine of infected persons; these people may have definite symptoms of the disease, or may be carriers as previously mentioned. Bad drainage systems and inefficient purification of drinking water can result in this being contaminated by excreta, and the infection is thus conveyed to others. In the UK the purification of most water supplies is so efficient as to make them safe for drinking purposes. *Food*, however, carries bacteria very readily, and certain foods (for example, reheated meat dishes and carelessly made ice-cream) provide a good medium in which bacteria may multiply. The typhoid organisms, and of course many others, may be conveyed to food by the hands of people who are either actively infected with disease or are carriers. This is a particularly insidious form of spread, as it may be difficult to find the source. For this reason it is important that those who handle food should make sure that after using a lavatory they wash their hands to exclude contamination by excreta.

(4) Insect carriage. Most of us are familiar with the fact that certain flying insects such as house-flies and blue bottles spread disease by conveying organisms, for example, from infected faeces to food. Parasites and vermin (for example, body lice and fleas) may also carry disease between people, and between animals and man. Malaria is conveyed to man by the bite of a particular mosquito which harbours the organisms.

Infection can be established in the body when bacteria have gained entry to it. They gain entry through a broken skin surface, and through natural orifices in the body such as the nose and mouth. Regions lined with mucous membrane give a warm moist environment which is favourable to bacterial growth.

Precautions are taken in hospital to prevent the spread of infection in any of the ways listed (see also Chapter 15). During surgery direct contact and aerial spread by droplet infection are the most likely ways for bacteria to be carried to the patient, and sterile techniques and sterilization of instruments and materials are methods of prevention unfailingly applied.

Bacteria are microscopic single-cell organisms, and they live, reproduce, and die. In order to live they require the following.

(1) Food – protein, carbohydrate, and mineral salts taken from tissue cells.
(2) Moisture.

(3) Oxygen. Some bacteria require air for their oxygen (*aerobic*), but others do not take it from the air, and in fact cannot live in air (*anaerobic*).

(4) An even temperature – 37°–38°C (98°–100°F).

(5) Generally an environment which is neither acid nor more than slightly alkaline and is unchanging.

The procedures used to achieve asepsis are directed to kill bacteria or prevent their growth by disturbance, in one way or another, of these conditions which they find favourable. Some bacteria discovering themselves in unfavourable conditions are able to achieve a phase of resistance, and such bacteria are called *spore-forming*. In this state they can resist some degree of heat, lack of moisture, cold, and the action of disinfectants.

In procedures for which aseptic precautions are required all the utensils, instruments, and materials for dressings will be sterilized. It must be remembered that such articles are not to be allowed to come in contact with others which have not been sterilized, and they must be handled with sterile forceps or by hands covered with sterile rubber gloves. The lightest touch of any non-sterile surface against one which *is* sterile contaminates the latter and invalidates its sterility. To ensure that this technique is correctly performed requires an undeviating attention to detail.

Methods of sterilization

Heat

Since heat kills all forms of bacteria it is the method of choice, unless it cannot be used because it will prove damaging to the article or material which is to be sterilized. In order to kill spore-forming bacteria it is necessary to achieve higher temperatures and longer periods of exposure than are lethal to the non-sporing type. In hospital practice, heat is used to sterilize as:

(1) Steam under pressure;

(2) Dry heat in an oven.

Sterilization by steam under pressure

Sterilization by steam under pressure is an efficient procedure. It is carried out in a piece of equipment called an autoclave. Articles put in an autoclave are subject to the action of steam at pressures above atmospheric pressure and temperatures above the boiling point of water (see Fig. 4.1).

In hospital, large autoclaves are found in sterilizing departments. Various materials are used to make a wrapping for articles to be autoclaved. Steam penetrates the wrapping, which yet provides (so long as it is intact and

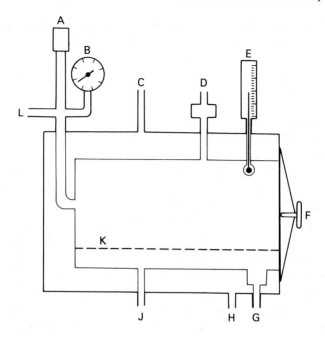

Fig. 4.1 Diagram showing a section through an autoclave. A safety valve; B pressure gauge; C steam inlet to jacket; D air inlet to chamber; E temperature gauge; F safety door; G chamber exhaust; H jacket exhaust; J steam extractor; K trivet; L steam inlet. *(Reproduced by courtesy of Churchill Livingstone and the College of Radiographers.)*

sealed) a covering through which the contents cannot be contaminated from the outside. In opening such a pack, care must be taken to see that only the outside edges and corners are handled, and that these are not subsequently allowed to fall against the inner parts of the wrapping to contaminate the contents (see Fig. 4.2).

Sterile packs should be handled as little as possible. All separate packs must bear outward evidence of sterilization, and this often takes the form of a special tape fastening the pack. The tape becomes striped after sterilization.

The hospital will use its autoclaving equipment as fully as possible, for it is not an economic procedure to bring it up to the required temperature and pressure, and hold it there for the necessary time unless the autoclave has a full load. The autoclaving process actually involves the loading of the autoclave, bringing it up to the correct temperature and pressure, and holding there for the required period. The time that this whole process needs depends upon several factors, the most important being the type of equipment in use. Modern high-pressure high vacuum equipment reaches higher temperatures more quickly, and sterilization is achieved in very much shorter times than would be possible with older apparatus. However,

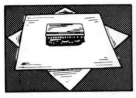
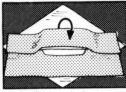
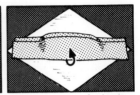

The contents of the pack – gauze, cotton wool, cellulose wadding etc. – are placed in a receiver in the centre of the *inner wrapper* which acts as the sterile area when the pack is opened for use. Underneath is the *outer protective* wrapper.

The *inner wrapper* is folded over in the manner shown so as to cover the contents.

The paper is again folded over so as to enclose the contents.

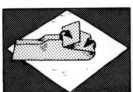
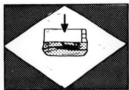
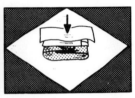

Both ends are neatly folded over the contents so that the wrapper can easily be opened when required.

The forceps in a paper bag or wrapper which will be used for opening the inner wrapper are then put on top.

A paper towel is put on top. This is for use as a sterile towel by the doctor or nurse who will be using the pack.

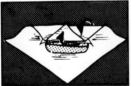
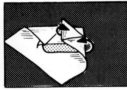
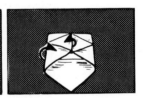

One corner of the *outer wrapper* is now folded over so as to cover the top of the contents and the corner folded back on top.

In a similar manner the paper is folded over to the centre of the pack and the corner turned back.

Fold the third corner over in a similar manner.

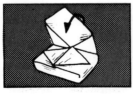
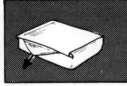
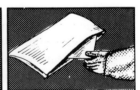

Then turn pack round and remaining flap of paper is folded over and tucked under the two top folds.

Leave the corner projecting out.

When the pack is ready to be used pull the corner out and open. The *outer wrapper* is opened by a person who need not be 'scrubbed up'.

Fig. 4.2 Illustration of the making of a sterile pack.

the time factor can be a problem when a busy clinic is sterilizing its own instruments in an autoclave installed in the clinic.

To check the efficacy of an autoclaving process, bacteriological tests can be carried out from time to time. Examples include the Bowie–Dick Test (Gunn & Jackson 1991) and the newer Lantor Cube test (3M Ltd., 1986).

Sterilization by dry heat

Moist heat is more penetrating and effective than dry heat (Bolding, 1988a), but hot dry air (or alternatively infra-red rays) can be used for efficient sterilization in an oven. In modern practice in sterilization departments, articles move slowly on a conveyer belt through an infra-red oven at a rate which brings them to the other end of their travel in a condition of sterility. The method is suitable for fragile glass ware such as test-tubes and syringes.

Gamma radiation

Gamma radiation, like heat, is a physical method of sterilization. Exposure to these electromagnetic radiations of very short wavelength is lethal to disease-producing organisms. It has the advantage that the penetrating character of the radiation enables it to be used to sterilize articles after they have been packaged; this makes it a valuable and commonly used method for manufacturers issuing pre-sterilized equipment. It may be used to sterilize articles which cannot be exposed to heat.

Chemical disinfection

Chemical disinfectants and antiseptics (which may be called weak disinfectants) have certain limitations in use. An efficient way of achieving *complete* sterility is to expose the organisms to a great enough heat for a long enough time, but obviously this is not possible with all materials and all equipment at all times. Chemical methods will then have to be used, although they are regarded as the least efficient choice.

It is important to recognize two separate actions which these chemicals may have. They may (1) kill bacteria (*bactericidal*) or (2) inhibit the growth of bacteria (*bacteriostatic*).

If it is desired to use a chemical agent to *kill* bacteria, it must be applied in greater strength and for a longer period of time than if the object is merely inhibition of growth.

There is no method of chemical sterilization which is completely effective in the sense that it will kill *all* organisms. *Spore-forming bacteria*, for example, withstand the action of chemical disinfectants more easily than that of heat. However, a reliable preparation used in sufficient strength for a long enough time can be expected to kill *most* organisms.

Articles put into disinfectant must be cleaned with soap and water before they go in, as the solution will be unable to act efficiently upon parts covered with organic matter such as mucus, pus, blood, etc. The container holding the disinfectant solution must itself be sterilized before the solution is put in, and there must be enough solution in it entirely to cover the articles which are to be disinfected. These must be totally immersed in it for the length of time required for the solution to act.

The particular agent used for any given purpose will depend upon various factors – whether the required effect is bacteriostatic or bactericidal, the nature of what is to be disinfected (for example surgical instruments, skin surfaces, linen, sluice room floors), and the practice of those who are using the agent.

Central sterile supply

Modern hospitals have central sterile supply services – a central department which supplies the hospital with all that is needed in ready sterilized equipment. This removes from the wards and special departments such as the X-ray department the need to sterilize items for their own use.

There are obvious advantages in such an arrangement which make it worth the financial outlay on instruments, washing equipment, and other specialized apparatus. It is less liable to failure in efficiency than a system which relies on separate sterilization processes carried out in many different places by different people with many demands on their time. A central department for sterilization where mechanization can be introduced and the efficacy of the whole system supervised must reduce the factor of human failure. Freed from the tasks of sterilizing equipment, we have more time to spend in the direct care of patients and on other aspects of what we do.

In order to use the central supply system, the ward or department in the hospital assesses its daily requirements of sterile equipment and receives this in suitable packs.

The modern tendency is towards making disposable as much of the equipment as can be so made, and applications of many modern materials are sought for this purpose. Aluminium foil, plastic, paper and cellulose are typical examples. Aluminium foil bowls, gallipots, and trays, paper dressing towels, and disposable hypodermic needles, syringes, and forceps are available, to be used once and then discarded. These provide an obvious saving in time and labour and an increase in the patient's safety.

In recent times such medical attention has been given to a serious risk to hospital staff which syringes and hypodermic needles may represent as conveyors of the virus of serum hepatitis (*jaundice*). This is a grave condition, much more severe than the milder infectious hepatitis for which a closely related virus is responsible. Deaths from the serum variety have occurred among workers in hospital who are occupationally concerned with procedures involving blood, the virus being carried in the blood of any patient who may once have had the disease. A far lesser risk, but one which has gained greater notoriety, is that of infection with the HIV virus (see also Chapter 15).

The availability of disposable equipment which is discarded as soon as it has been used does much to limit the risk but student radiographers and anyone who may have to handle syringes and needles should recognize the danger and exercise care to avoid being pricked. Once used, a needle must **never** be resheathed and must be placed in the sharps box provided.

Preparation of the hands for aseptic procedures

It has long been the practice of surgeons and nurses to prepare their hands by 'scrubbing up' – thoroughly washing and scrubbing the hands with warm water, soap, and nail brush for a period of 5 to 10 minutes, usually with the use of bacteriostatic soap or suitable antiseptic solution. It seems to be open to debate among surgeons as to whether this process renders the hands sterile or just clean, but the safest and most regular procedure is to consider that the hands are not in fact sterile and cannot be put in contact with sterilized materials. In any case, whichever view a particular surgeon may hold, his practice will be to enclose his hands in sterile rubber gloves before he handles sterilized instruments, and anyone who assists him and also directly handles sterilized materials will do the same. The correct technique for putting on sterile gloves is shown in Fig. 4.3. It is now thought that it may be possible to replace the 'scrubbing up' process by a less time-consuming technique of immersion of the hands in suitable solutions of centrimide and chlorhexidine.

Certain procedures such as surgical dressings are carried out with what is called the 'no touch' technique, all the dressing requirements which are sterile being manipulated with sterile forceps and not touched by hand. In this technique it is unnecessary to try to achieve sterility of the hands, and it is a safe procedure just to wash the hands well in soap and water and dry them on a clean towel. In modern practice the towel is a paper one, used once and then discarded.

Laying up a sterile trolley

Detailed requirements in setting up trays or trolleys for sterile procedures will clearly depend on the nature of the treatment or examination for which

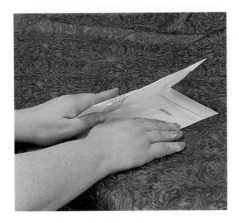

(a) Opening packet.

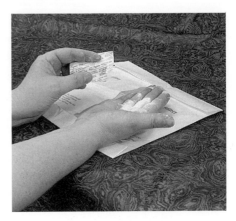

(b) Powdering hands.

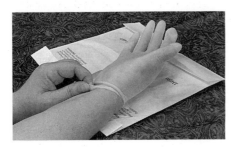

(c) Inserting first hand, holding by inside of cuff only.

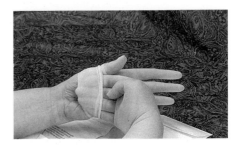

(d) Inserting second hand; glove on first hand in contact with outside of second glove.

Fig. 4.3 Showing correct method of putting on sterile gloves.

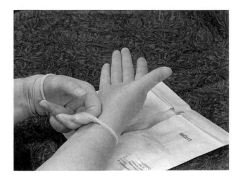 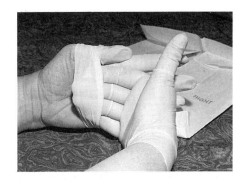

(e) Turning back first cuff.   (f) Turning back second cuff.

the equipment is being prepared. Certain principles of technique, however, are basic and common to many procedures, and should be understood if conditions of asepsis are to be preserved.

It is a general rule that when a trolley is being laid up with both sterile and unsterile equipment, the top shelf is reserved as the sterile field, while the lower shelf holds unsterile accessories. It may be assumed that in common practice the procedure for which the trolley is prepared will be undertaken by means of prepared packs from a central sterile supply department. In this case, typical items for the lower shelf would be the required pack, an antiseptic spray for cleaning the trolley, a skin cleanser, adhesive strapping and a pair of scissors. Used items (for example, dressings, swabs, disposable instruments) are discarded nowadays into paper bags. Sharp things such as disposable scalpels and needles which can penetrate a soft wrapping are discarded into special containers which will not readily puncture and can be firmly closed. The containers are labelled for the reception of discarded 'sharps'. The paper bags are clipped to the sides of the trolley with 'bulldog' clips or plastic clothes-pegs, the one for used instruments on the left side, and the soiled dressings bag on the right. After use, the top of the dressings bag is closed with a twist, and it is put in the dirty-dressings bin for incineration. The instruments are either discarded or are returned to a central sterile supply according to the practice of the hospital.

The hands are always to be considered as non-sterile unless they are in sterile rubber gloves, and they therefore must not come in contact with any sterile material. Before preparing for or undertaking a sterile procedure, the hands must be properly washed with warm water and soap, and well dried upon a disposable paper towel; wet articles and wet areas favour the spread of bacteria.

People concerned in sterile procedures and in handling sterile equipment should wear masks, although it is not generally the custom to do this when the procedure being undertaken is a simple intravenous injection. The mask covers both mouth and nose and is made of layers of muslin, often with a sheet of cellophane inserted between the layers. The upper edge of the mask may be stiffened with a little curved metal strip to hold it firmly against the nose. The cellophane makes the front of the mask impervious to the moisture produced by respiration; a wet mask will be an inadequate barrier against droplet infection from the nose and mouth of the wearer. Disposable masks of paper are available, but these must not be worn for periods longer than 10 minutes as they are penetrable by moisture eventually. In some hospitals, nurses no longer wear masks when doing a round of dressings because in these circumstances paper masks are worn too long to be of any help.

It is recognized that any face mask, however good, is not a perfect barrier and organisms will evade it at its edges. Furthermore if a mask is not properly handled on removal it can cause more trouble than its use may be expected to prevent. The correct technique is to remove the mask by handling only the tapes or bands which attach it to the head and then at once to discard it. In practice a wearer may just pull it down, in the process transferring to the hands organisms from the front of the mask. Instead of being discarded, the mask is worn for a while around the neck or is removed and stuffed into a pocket; both these malpractices easily transfer organisms to the clothes.

Because of these facts, in some places the use of a face mask is being discontinued even in operating theatres. In these circumstances regular throat swabs are taken from the staff to make sure that they are not carrying pathogenic organisms. The presence of these would of course make the droplets discharged from nose and mouth especially unwholesome.

A simple sterile dressing

Surgical dressings of operation wounds and burns (the latter are considered to be particularly liable to infection) are undertaken in the wards in controlled conditions of asepsis. It is most unlikely that a radiographer in the diagnostic X-ray department will be called upon to deal with a major dressing. If a patient comes to the department with a dressing in place which contains radiopaque elements such as 'Elastoplast' or jaconet, it should not be summarily removed. Advice should be sought from the ward or department from which the patient has been referred concerning the removal of such a dressing and its possible replacement.

If the patient comes to the department with a surgical dressing in place which during the course of the examination becomes dislodged, or becomes wet with blood or other discharge from the wound, fresh sterile dressings should be applied to cover the previous one, and the ward or department referring the patient should be told of the occurrence.

Undertaking a simple sterile dressing *may* come within the province of a radiographer, and it should be understood that the important principle to be observed in doing it is the maintenance of asepsis by correct sterile technique. A trolley must be prepared, reference being made to the precautions described previously. The requirements for the trolley are the following.

Upper shelf – sterile area

- The trolley surfaces and legs are cleaned using an antiseptic aerosol spray.
- They are dried with a paper towel.
- The clean trolley-top will be used for setting up a sterile area from which the dressing will be done.

Lower shelf – non-sterile area

The lower shelf of the trolley should have available upon it:

- A medium dressing pack or basic dressing pack from the central sterile supply department;
- Some adhesive strapping;
- A skin cleansing lotion such as chlorhexidine, 0.05% in aqueous solution;
- A face mask if it is to be worn;
- A pair of scissors of the surgical type (that is, with rounded ends to the blades);
- Sometimes an extra pair of presterilized dissecting forceps in a container;
- Sometimes a skin anaesthetic in an aerosol spray.

Two paper bags are attached to the trolley, one for instruments on the left side and the soiled dressings bag on the right side. Sometimes one bag only is used for both.

The technique employed is described as a *no touch technique*, and this means that the hands do not touch any part of the wound or the area round the wound, or any material which will be applied directly to the wound. The dressing must be managed with sterile forceps. If this cannot be done sterile rubber gloves must be worn; it is here assumed that the straightforward type of dressing most likely to be encountered in the diagnostic X-ray department can be managed with forceps alone.

Before the dressing is begun the patient should be placed in such a position that the area to be dressed is horizontal. When this is so, dressings can be laid in place without risk of their falling off, and it will not be necessary to hold them in place with forceps while outer dressings are applied.

The hands of the person undertaking the procedure should be preserved from contact with grossly contaminated material such as soiled dressings. The outer dressings may be removed by hand, but the inner ones should be lifted away with forceps (Kelso, 1989).

Fig. 4.4 shows a technique to be used for a basic dressing by means of presterilized prepared packs. From this it can be seen that typical contents of a basic dressing pack are as follows:

- Four pairs of dissecting forceps;
- Four cotton wool balls;
- Three gauze squares;
- Two aluminium foil gallipots;
- One large clinical sheet.

The top of the trolley is left entirely clear. The lower shelf holds:

(1) The sterile pack;
(2) Brown paper bags and pegs;
(3) Accessories such as masks, bandages, pins, adhesive strapping, and a pair of scissors;
(4) A skin cleansing agent;
(5) A pair of dissecting forceps (sterile) in a separate container.

It will be possible to open the pack without touching any part other than the outside, and the inner wrapping can be spread out to form a sterile field on top of the trolley (see Fig. 4.4).

There will usually be two layers of wrapping, the outer one perhaps being a paper bag. This outer layer can be removed after the hands have been washed and a mask (if worn) put on at the start of the dressing technique. When the inner wrapping is spread out to cover the trolley top, the dressings and gallipot are lying directly on it.

As shown in Fig. 4.4, the large dissecting forceps are dropped from the container into the hand (the points not being touched). They are then used to arrange the contents of the pack.

The dressing is undertaken with a 'no touch technique', as described. It will be necessary to lift the dissecting forceps by hand from the trolley top. Care should be taken to touch only the handles and not the points of any of the forceps.

In ward practice it is necessary to clean a wound when the dressing is changed. However, as this is a technique which is infrequently undertaken by radiographers it is probably best practice to clean only around the wound

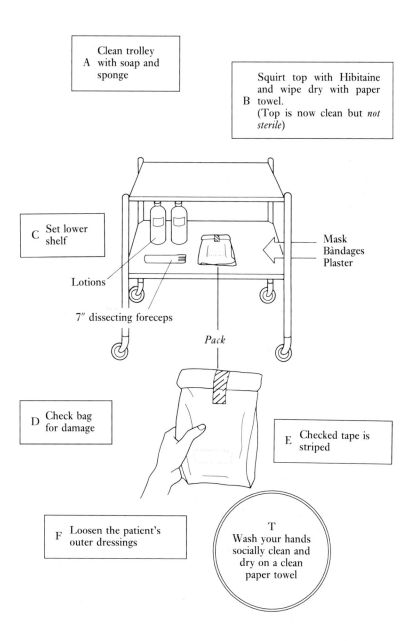

Fig. 4.4 Basic dressing technique using sterile packs. *(Prepared in conjunction with Guy's Hospital and reproduced by kind permission of Guy's Hospital and the Bowater-Scott Corporation Ltd.)*

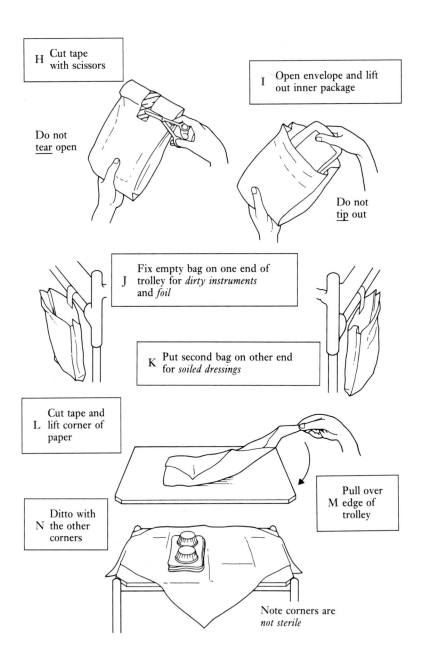

H Cut tape with scissors

Do not tear open

I Open envelope and lift out inner package

Do not tip out

J Fix empty bag on one end of trolley for *dirty instruments* and *foil*

K Put second bag on other end for *soiled dressings*

L Cut tape and lift corner of paper

M Pull over edge of trolley

N Ditto with the other corners

Note corners are *not sterile*

Fig. 4.4 *cont.*

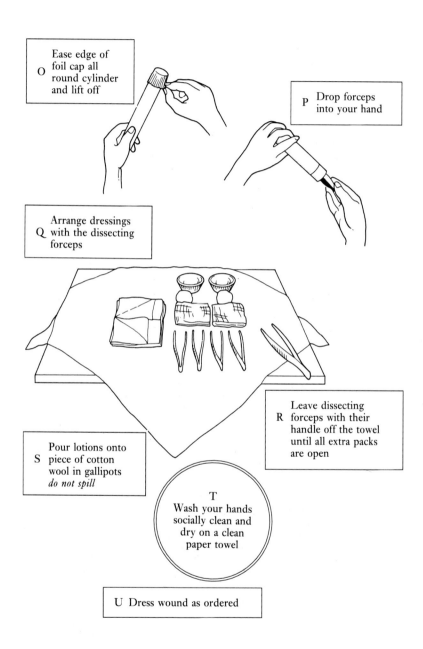

O Ease edge of foil cap all round cylinder and lift off

P Drop forceps into your hand

Q Arrange dressings with the dissecting forceps

R Leave dissecting forceps with their handle off the towel until all extra packs are open

S Pour lotions onto piece of cotton wool in gallipots *do not spill*

T Wash your hands socially clean and dry on a clean paper towel

U Dress wound as ordered

Fig. 4.4 *cont.*

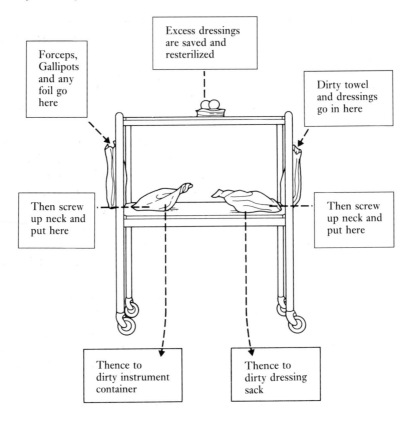

Forceps,
Gallipots
and any
foil go
here

Excess dressings
are saved and
resterilized

Dirty towel
and dressings
go in here

Then screw
up neck and
put here

Then screw
up neck and
put here

Thence to
dirty instrument
container

Thence to
dirty dressing
sack

Fig. 4.4 *cont.*

or, if the wound itself appears to *need* cleaning, ask a member of nursing staff to undertake the procedure. There is conflicting advice regarding methods of cleaning the wound itself and lack of care may lead to wound contamination. Many departments now have their own nursing staff, who will be more practised in this technique and able to carry it out quickly and safely. To clean around the wound you take a pair of forceps in each hand, pick up a cotton wool ball with one pair of forceps, soak the ball in the skin lotion and then squeeze out the surplus fluid by means of the other pair of forceps. Each swab should be used for one stroke only and is discarded as soon as it is lifted from the skin. Keep discarding the used swabs into the disposable bag attached to the trolley.

If at any time it is necessary to replace forceps on the trolley *after* they have been handled but *without* having had their points contaminated by contact with unsterile material it is very important that they should be placed with the points inwards to rest within (while the handles are outside) the defined boundary of the sterile area. This placing can be seen for the large forceps in Fig. 4.4.

After cleansing, the wound is dried with sterile cotton wool balls. Finally the wound is dressed by using forceps to place the gauze over it to give complete cover. Strapping is applied to keep the dressing firmly and comfortably in place.

When the dressing is finished, the gallipots, paper wrappings, etc., are discarded into the soiled-dressings bag on the side of the trolley, and the forceps are put into the soiled-forceps container for eventual return to the central sterile supply department.

A modern technique for ward dressings has been introduced in some hospitals in the United Kingdom. Complete dressing packs, sealed and sterilized by the manufacturer, are used. This is called a pre-set tray system and each pack contains equipment for a dressing (including wound-cleansing lotion in a plastic sachet) and a fresh pack is used for each patient. The contents are packed in a plastic tray with moulded gallipots as a part of it, and the tray acts as a sterile field while the dressing is being done. Everything, from the tray itself to the plastic and metal forceps, is disposable.

The pack is sealed within an air-tight and water-tight polythene covering and is sterilized by radiation before it leaves the manufacturer. These commercial packs are supplied under strict controls and provide a standardized sterile dressing which should be of great help in reducing cross-infection in all hospitals, from the largest to the smallest, where they are used.

References

Bolding, B. (1988a) Steam sterilisation systems: how they work (Part 1). *Canadian Operating Room Nursing Journal*, 6 (3), 9–12.

Bolding, B. (1988b) Steam sterilisation systems; safety and proper processing (part 2). *Canadian Operating Room Nursing Journal*, 6 (6), 28–32.

Gunn, C. & Jackson, C.S. (1991) *Guidelines on Patient Care in Radiography*, (page 54), 2nd Edn., Churchill Livingstone, Edinburgh.

Kelso, H. (1989) Alternative technique. *Nursing times*, 85 (23), 70–72.

3M Ltd (1986) *New Test System for Autoclaves*. Press release; Loughborough 3M Health Care Ltd.

Chapter 5
Preparation of the Patient

Introduction to general aspects of patient preparation

It is wise to regard nearly all X-ray examinations as requiring some preparation of the patient. Before discussing the gastrointestinal tract specifically, we shall examine the principles of patient preparation. Firstly let us consider *physical* preparation; in the strict sense of the term preparation of the patient has been made when merely a jacket or frock is removed prior to the X-ray examination of a limb. This is a simple procedure. More elaborate preliminaries are required for many investigations with which the student will become familiar, for example, prior to radiography of the abdomen.

Physical preparation of a patient is important if we are to reduce the need for repeat examinations. This may be the local preparation of a part or it may be the general preparation of a system; the alimentary, the urinary or other tracts. It may be undertaken immediately prior to the X-ray examination, as mentioned above, or it may extend over 2 or even 3 days and require the administration of certain medicines and drugs.

In relation to the appropriate preparation of patients who are to have X-ray examinations the responsibilities of the radiographer are broadly two-fold. In the first place it should be made clear to the patient what is required of them and, if they are to attend for the examination at a later date, this must include some indication of the length of time the procedure is likely to occupy.

Like ourselves many of our patients lead busy lives. The mother of a family may require to make special arrangements for the care of young children in her absence; the businessman probably has a full schedule of engagements. It is most unfair to allow either of these to attend the X-ray department believing that it is a matter of no more than a few minutes, when in fact the significant procedure is more likely to occupy up to 2 hours. To the radiographer such features of any examination are so familiar that it is very easy to overlook their strangeness to the patient. The omission of that moment or two of sympathetic explanation may at the time seem trivial to the radiographer, but such matters can add significantly to the patient's anxiety about the examination. This brings us to the second component of patient preparation: psychological preparation. We must remember that examinations which we as radiographers take for granted can be very traumatic for patients. The Patient's Charter now gives patients a right to information about their care and it is important to give the patient a full explanation of the procedure they will undergo and to take time to deal with any worries they may express about what will happen to them. It is also necessary to realize that patients 'fill in the gaps'; in other words, if we don't tell them what is to happen they will make their own assumptions, which will often be far worse than the reality! Radiographers have a responsibility to reduce patient anxiety wherever possible; this in turn will reduce the need for repeat exposures and thus keep radiation dose as low as possible.

The responsibilities of the radiographer, if in the first place to the patients themselves, are secondly to those others in the hospital who have patients in their immediate care. In an earlier chapter observation has been made of the close inter-relationship of members of the medical team. No department, no unit within the hospital can properly be considered as an isolated entity. We are all interdependent. We cannot provide our best service for the patient if others in the hospital do not know something of what we are trying to do or understand the way in which it may be done.

To this end it is clearly essential that we should keep ward and departmental sisters conversant with our requirements for the preparation of all patients. We should see that this information is given accurately and that it is kept up to date.

Such preparation is not absolute and universal. It will vary in detail between hospitals, due to the individual methods and requirements of each consultant radiologist. Even in any one hospital, it will and should undergo variation in the course of time. All branches of medicine are continuously advancing; discoveries are made, a fresh conception arises and a new practice is introduced.

It is a straightforward matter in any X-ray department to have duplicated sheets of simple instructions relating to the preparation of patients for X-ray examination, whether these be special procedures or even plain investigations requiring only immediate preliminaries. All wards and departments can then be circularized with this information and in the same way notified of changes as these become necessary. It is important to keep all facts issued – in whatever form – fully up to date.

General abdominal preparation

Many diagnostic imaging examinations involve the visualization of abdominal organs, for example intravenous urography and barium meal. Whatever may be the special preparation required for each procedure, they have in common the feature that difficulties of interpretation sometimes arise because of confusing shadows in the lower alimentary tract, due to the normal presence of faeces and intestinal gas. Bowel preparation has custo-marily been used for all such examinations in the past, but some radiologists are now sceptical about the efficacy of the use of purgatives. For example, bowel cramps caused by some preparations may cause the patient to swallow air, thus producing excessive bowel gas. In some departments, therefore, the use of purgatives for examinations such as intravenous urography has been abandoned. Equally, those laxatives that are available are now deemed to be so effective that the use of enemata for the preparation of patients has been almost universally abandoned.

Use of purgatives

Usually preparation begins with the administration of the drug 48 to 36 hours or in some cases 24 hours before the examination. In certain condi-tions, however, the taking of any such drug is contra-indicated, for example in the presence of diarrhoea, haemorrhage or obstruction. In the case of in-patients any drug used will be given under nursing supervision on the ward. However, where outpatients are concerned it is the radiographer's responsibility to ensure that the patient receives proper instruction.

If purgatives are to be classified it is logical to consider differences between them in the ways they act. They may be divided into three groups:

(1) Irritant purgatives;
(2) Lubricant purgatives;
(3) Bulk purgatives.

Irritant purgatives

The method of action of the so-called irritant purgatives is not fully understood and the term 'irritant' is perhaps misleading: certainly it over-simplifies, since all the drugs in this group do not act in exactly the same way. The following substances are examples of irritant purgatives.

Bisacodyl (*'Dulcolax'*) and *Picolax* (now commonly used in X-ray departments) both produce peristalsis (automatic wavelike contractions) of the gut – mainly the large bowel – on contact with the mucous membrane which lines it; they have an irritant effect upon the sensory nerve endings in the mucosa. Administration may be either oral, in tablet form, or by means of a suppository inserted at the anus.

Senna and *cascara* are both vegetable purgatives and are similar in their action, which is thought to be direct stimulation of a plexus of automatic nerves (Auerbach's plexus) between the muscular coats of the bowel.

Lubricant purgatives

The operation of lubricant purgatives by softening faeces is easy to understand.

Also in this group is a substance, *dioctylsodium sulphosuccinate* which lubricates the faeces by lowering surface tension and permitting water to penetrate them: compare the function of a photographic wetting agent in promoting the effective action of developer upon a film emulsion. '*Normax*' is an example of a purgative which contains dioctylsodium sulphosuccinate as one of its active ingredients.

Bulk purgatives
Bulk purgatives achieve their purpose – generally in one to three hours after administration – by increasing the volume of intestinal contents: the result is to stretch the bowel wall and encourage normal peristaltic activity.

The drugs in this group obtain the same effect in one of two different ways.

(1) The important active ingredient is an indigestible plant material (methyl cellulose, psyllium seed and sterculia are examples) or vegetable fibre which absorbs water in the intestine and swells.
(2) The active substance is an inorganic salt which is not absorbable and by a process of osmosis retains water in the lumen of the bowel. Osmosis is the tendency of fluids which are different in concentration and separated by a permeable membrane – in this case the bowel wall – to mix with each other, the solvent of the solution which is less in concentration passing into the solution of higher concentration.

'*Celevac*', '*Isogel*' and '*Normacol X*' are examples of bulk-forming evacuants of the first type; Epsom salts (magnesium sulphate) is a well-known member of the saline group.

Side effects of purgatives
The side effects of purgatives are numerous and varied and occasionally have been fatal. Some, usually elderly people, may dose themselves regularly with a purgative in large quantities and without any medical advice over a long period of time: they may suffer from such consequences as electrolyte deficiency and protein loss. Sometimes the indiscriminate self-administration of a purgative has masked a serious condition, such as acute appendicitis, with tragic results. It is well for us to remember, whenever we instruct a patient to take a laxative prior to X-ray examination, that we are giving a potentially harmful drug.

Lower abdominal discomfort, flatulence and colic may not be particularly serious but are now extremely common side effects of purgation, particularly where the newer agents such as *Picolax* or *X-Prep* are employed. Almost inevitably for some patients disagreeable side effects – of pain, spasm and severe diarrhoea – will occur.

Because so many aperients are in some degree unpredictable and inconstant in action it is difficult to formulate an ideal preparation for abdominal radiography. Departmental routines are developed from the preferences of the radiologist in charge who will have selected in the course of his experience some one method from several which are reasonably satisfactory; or a medicine may be chosen which has been formulated solely for use in radiographic abdominal preparation, such as *Picolax*. It is the radiographer's responsibility to be familiar in detail with the method in departmental use and to ensure that the out patient receives correct instruction in its application.

On this point of instruction of the patient some further observations should be made. Many patients attending hospital will accept incuriously and with unquestioning placidity anything which they are given and directed to take. If the radiographer is busy and suffering from the pressure of several other people who require attention, it is likely that the assumption will be made that the patient understands what they are receiving and – as they do not ask about it – that they know the effect it will have. In many instances this is far from being the case.

No outpatient should be instructed to take an aperient given to him, without at the same time being informed of its nature. This is important in the administration of any drug, and not least in this procedure which may appear relatively insignificant to the busy radiographer. It is most undesirable, and even cruel, to issue a standard dose of some aperient to all patients. Obviously their individual needs in this respect will vary, and very often patients themselves are the best judge of the doses they should take.

Before being given the medicine each patient should be questioned a little about their normal bowel habits. Where appropriate, further advice should be sought before sending the patient the aperient.

Young patients require special consideration. If strong purgation is to be avoided in adults, it is particularly undesirable in the case of a child. Children under a year of age should not be given an aperient and some paediatricians may not regard with favour the routine preparation of their patients for X-ray examination. If a bowel evacuant is considered necessary it may be better to rely on whatever aperient the mother normally uses for the child when need arises. The suppository form of bisacodyl already mentioned is also useful as *one* can safely be given to a child over 12 months of age. It is small enough to be easily inserted even in a youngster.

Prevention of intestinal gas

It has been earlier stated that the presence of intestinal gas can seriously impair radiographic detail and may delay diagnosis. It is in fact often a more troublesome problem than faecal residues. For example, a common difficulty in cholecystography is the superimposition upon the opacified gall bladder of radiolucencies which may be either gall stones or pockets of gas in the small or large bowel.

Some pathological conditions give rise to abnormal gas shadows on the radiograph. For example, air may be seen to have leaked outside the alimentary tract in the case of a perforated gastric ulcer; or gas may accumulate massively and distend the bowel proximal to the site of an intestinal obstruction. In these instances its appearance is helpful to diagnosis and indeed may considerably influence treatment.

In any random group of people, nearly all would be found to have gas present to some degree in the stomach and in the lower alimentary tract. Certain circumstances favour its collection. *Diet*, for example, is a factor. The subject may be eating starchy foods (carbohydrates) or vegetables such as parsnips, peas or beans, which tend to produce gas during digestion: or they may be addicted to effervescent drinks. Again, they may be an '*air swallower*', a nervous habit likely to become accentuated under the slight tension of a visit to hospital and an impending X-ray examination. Confinement to bed is also a significant factor, as during prolonged *immobility* intestinal gas is less readily absorbed or dispersed. Adequate preparation is aimed at reducing the amount likely to be present in any individual by avoiding, whenever possible, those circumstances which increase or are favourable to its formation.

To this end a very simple but important measure is to include in the department's instructions to nursing and other hospital staff a request that any patient who is sufficiently fit should be out of bed at least for part of the day prior to the examination, or even only for an hour or so immediately before coming to the department. However, in many cases it is impossible for the patient to be on his feet and then it may unfortunately be a matter of trying to effect the absorption of accumulated gas which the patient is unable to disperse. In this case there are certain recognized treatments which may be helpful. These include:

(1) The use of a flatus tube;
(2) The giving of one or two charcoal biscuits to eat at bed-time on the night prior to the X-ray examination.

As has been noted, diet is a significant factor and some attention should be paid to this during the 48 hours prior to examination. On the day prior to the examination the patient may be advised to take a *low residue diet*, avoiding green vegetables, cereals and wholemeal bread. On the morning of the examination itself, if this is to be a simple radiograph of the urinary or biliary tract, it is usual to allow the patient to take a light breakfast. Some radiologists prefer that nothing should be taken from the previous midnight and in this case it should be noted that if the patient is to come starving to the department special considerations apply to the diabetic subject. This will be more fully studied in Chapter 6.

Chapter 6
The Gastrointestinal Tract

Radiological investigations of the gastrointestinal tract, by barium meal and barium enema, are still very frequently performed. In any general X-ray department these procedures may constitute a large section of the week's work and occupy one or more X-ray rooms for a considerable part of any day or days set aside for the purpose. Since a fluoroscopic examination by a radiologist is an essential feature of these procedures it is usual to arrange for the radiologist to see a series of patients referred at one time; the radiologist will undertake a 'screening' session on a morning or afternoon suitable to him/her and to the department.

The number of cases likely to be examined during any one session will vary widely, depending on local features. The availability of radiological staff, the radiologist's own assessment of the number of patients that can be properly examined at one time, the size of the department and the pressure of work on it, are all among significant factors in determining the number of appointments which may be made.

It is customary to divide each session into cases for examination by barium meal (including barium swallow) and those for examination by barium enema. Alternatively separate sessions may be set aside for each.

The separation of the meal and enema bookings is important from the point of view of saving time, facilitating work and promoting hygiene. Each type of examination needs its own minor specialized equipment: for example, the trolley lay-out.

If it is properly used it is a recognized advantage of any appointment system that waiting time can be appreciably decreased. In 'block booking' patients for gastrointestinal examination some attention should be paid to the length of time likely to be required for each case. It is not a proper use of the system if the last patient to be examined has been told to come at the same hour and minute as the first. Not only is this discourteous to patients, but it should also now be seen as contravening the spirit of the Patient's Charter.

It is likely that the time allowed for each examination will be underestimated, whereas the likelihood that some patients will fail to attend may be overestimated. All these of course are important considerations. Those responsible for the allocation of appointments should try to evaluate them reasonably and reach a balance which will be acceptable as a working system.

In this and in succeeding chapters each special radiological procedure will be discussed under three similar headings.

(1) Specific preparation of the patient.
(2) Preparation and management of the examination.
(3) Care of the patient

Barium meal: barium swallow

Preparation of the patient

In the previous chapter reference was made to some general points. These include:

(1) Indication to the patient of the amount of time likely to be required for (*a*) the initial fluoroscopic examination, and (*b*) any follow-through series of films which may be suggested on the request form or which may be customary in the department;
(2) Such instruction as is routine in the department in relation to general preparation for abdominal radiography.

The alimentary tract is not inherently opaque to X-rays and cannot therefore be directly examined. It becomes opaque upon the introduction of a suitable contrast agent, barium sulphate, which fills the lumen of the tract and thereby will reveal irregularities due to pathology: for example, ulceration, neoplasia, or constrictive lesions.

The radiological appearances can be reliable only if the stomach is empty at the time the meal is taken. A misleading impression of deformity may be received if the barium pattern is distorted by the presence of food residues.

Because of these physical principles it is essential that no patient who is to have a barium meal should come to the X-ray department having recently taken either food or drink. It is important that instructions on this point should be specific: a patient told not to eat may well think that the restriction does not apply to a glass of milk or an early morning cup of tea. It is usual, if the X-ray examination is to be in the morning, to instruct the patient to take nothing by mouth after the evening meal on the previous night. This probably means that he has eaten last some 12 or 15 hours prior to taking the barium meal and of course this is a starvation period of more than adequate margin.

The diabetic patient

In any preparation involving restriction of diet, special attention must be paid to the diabetic subject.

There are two types of diabetes.

(1) *Diabetes mellitus*, which is due to deficiency of insulin secretion by the pancreas. There may be partial or complete failure of secretion. Diabetes mellitus is relatively common and is the most common of the metabolic diseases.
(2) *Diabetes insipidus*, which arises from impaired function of the posterior lobe of the pituitary gland. This is a *very rare* condition.

Insulin is a secretion of the islets of Langerhans in the pancreas. Its function in the blood stream is to control the reserve of sugar which is stored in liver and muscle in the form of glycogen A failure in supply of insulin immediately raises the level of blood sugar and this condition is known as *hyperglycaemia*. Sugar appears also in the urine (*glycosuria*).

A disturbance of sugar metabolism in the body is associated with impaired combustion of fats, as the one process assists the other. When the oxidation of fats is only partial, certain aceto-acetic acids or *ketones* are formed in the blood. This condition is known as *ketosis* and leads to hyperglycaemia in the untreated subject.

Diabetes mellitus is not curable and must be treated by initial hospitalization where the patient is stabilized and taught to recognize the individual symptoms of *hypoglycaemia*.

Long-term management of the disease is by:

(1) Correct diet, maintaining a balance of carbohydrate and fat, and of proper calorific value;
(2) Insulin administration in all but mature onset diabetes which may be managed by diet and an oral hypoglycaemic agent.

With this treatment the blood sugar can be kept at normal level, the patient is free of glycosuria, and their diabetes is said to be stabilized. Once a proper balance has been found, it is clearly of some significance that there should be little interference with the diet. Anyone known to be a diabetic must receive proper instruction if it becomes necessary for that person to omit or limit a normal meal.

The patient should be told to omit breakfast *and* the insulin injection, but must be placed *first* on the morning's list for examination, and the radiographer is responsible for ensuring that the patient in fact receives attention quickly. If wishing to bring their own food patients should, on completion of the X-ray examination, be allowed privacy, away from other patients and general departmental traffic. If food has not been brought, a sandwich or similar may be obtained on the patient's behalf from the hospital canteen.

Hyper-and hypoglycaemia

Two forms of unconsciousness are associated with diabetes:

(1) Hyperglycaemia (diabetic coma);
(2) Hypoglycaemia (insulin coma).

Should a diabetic subject become unconscious while in the X-ray department it may be of importance that the radiographer is able to recognize each type of coma. Rapidity of onset is a significant point: a diabetic patient, apparently normal on arrival, who subsequently becomes faint or unconscious, is almost certainly suffering from hypoglycaemia. The signs of both types of coma, however, are given below.

Diabetic coma (hyperglycaemia)

The first occurs in a subject in whom the disease is untreated or from whom the correct dose of insulin has been for some reason withheld. It is due, as has been explained already, to the accumulation in the blood of aceto-acetic acids through faulty combustion of fats. It is of slow onset, taking as a rule a matter of days to develop.

(1) Drowsiness and eventual unconsciousness;
(2) Stertorous deep breathing. (The respiratory centre is stimulated and endeavours to restore via the lungs the normal chemical balance of the body.)
(3) A sweet smell of acetone on the breath.
(4) A dry skin.

This patient requires insulin by hypodermic injection and urgent medical attention.

Insulin coma (hypoglycaemia)

Insulin coma, on the other hand, may occur in a patient who has received too much insulin. This may be because the dose has been wrongly given, or equally it may arise in a patient who has taken the correct amount of insulin but has not eaten food, so that he has little sugar on which the insulin can work. His blood sugar falls to an abnormally low level (*hypoglycaemia*) and unconsciousness results. It is of rapid onset and may develop within an hour of the patient's arrival at the hospital.

(1) A sinking feeling, accompanied by hunger.
(2) Faintness and eventual unconsciousness.
(3) Quiet shallow breathing.
(4) Absence of the characteristic breath odour.
(5) Sweating and moist clammy skin.

This patient requires glucose. Its administration must be intravenous if unconsciousness is complete. In some cases an injection of glucagon or adrenaline may be made. Either of these releases the patient's own reserves of 'sugar' stored as glycogen in the liver. However, if the patient is able to take anything by mouth a can of fizzy, sugary drink should be administered. This dissolves quickly through the lining of the stomach into the blood-stream.

Preparation of infants for barium swallow/meal

The procedure to be followed in the case of babies who are to have a barium meal requires some notice. Usually the child is being fed four hourly. The mother may give the customary meal at 6.0 AM but should not feed the child again until after completion of the X-ray examination. This will ensure firstly that the stomach is empty and secondly that the patient is hungry on arrival in the X-ray department, no small factor in the successful admin-istration of an unusual drink in unusual surroundings. It is wise to give the mother a word of explanation as to the reason for the starvation; otherwise, if the baby becomes fretful and crying through hunger, she may be tempted to feed it before coming to the hospital. The X-ray examination should be timed for 10.0 AM or as near to that hour as possible.

It has sometimes been advocated that the barium sulphate mixture should be mixed in suitable quantity with the child's customary food and the two given in combination: the principle presumably is that the child will accept such a mixture more readily. However, the system has little to recommend it. The fat present in milk leads to flocculation of the barium sulphate and visualization of the alimentary tract is impaired. Secondly the combination of barium sulphate and water with the dried milk powder usually employed often seems to result in a thickly viscous consistency, more solid than fluid, which the patient cannot take.

A preferable method is to replace the child's 10 AM feed with a normally prepared barium drink administered in a feeding bottle of conventional type. A baby who is hungry will generally show little reluctance to take it.

The most difficult patient is the toddler who has to be persuaded to drink from a cup an unusual drink which, even if he is hungry, he will probably find that he does not like. The toddler's mother or father, if present, may or may not prove an asset to the radiographer. Sometimes in these circum-stances children are found to respond better to the ministrations of a stranger with whom there is no emotional link, but it is as well for the radiographer to discover from the parents as much as possible about the child.

The correct use of a name or nickname is an obvious beginning. If the child enjoys drinking through a straw, allowing the barium to be taken in this way may be adequate encouragement. If the youngster is averse to milk, the appearance of the barium sulphate will be off-putting at the start, and in this case a suitable colouring agent might well be added.

Preparation and management of the examination

Before the beginning of each fluoroscopic list a 'barium trolley' should be made ready containing all that will be needed for the complete session of 'meals'. A 'barium preparation' room is a feature of many departments. Here barium contrast agents and their accessories can be stored and made ready in accordance with the requirements of the radiologist concerned and poured ready for use into the appropriate number of beakers or tumblers set ready on a tray. A number of proprietary preparations of barium sulphate are available. Barium sulphate is insoluble in water and will be given to the patient as a liquid suspension. Sometimes this is the form in which the manufacturer supplies it; but also employed are powdered barium preparations, to which the user must add water in accordance with the instructions of the manufacturer. When it is ready, the mixture preferred for the usual double contrast study combines a high concentration of barium sulphate with low viscosity. These characteristics mean that the contrast agent:

(1) Can freely coat – and thus delineate fully – the mucosae of the alimentary tract;
(2) Will flow readily in the gastrointestinal tract and is easily taken by mouth.

A typical presentation of a high density barium sulphate consists of a closed tumbler-shaped carton (500 ml capacity) containing 312 g of barium sulphate powder (96% w/w barium sulphate). To this the radiographer adds 83 ml of water; and then – having replaced the cap firmly! – shakes the assembly briskly for about a minute to obtain adequate dispersion of the powder. Further shaking should be given immediately before administration to a patient. The result is 150 ml of 200% w/v barium sulphate suspension. Other high density barium sulphates are similar, although not identical to this; for instance the final suspension may be 250% w/v.

A different, well known barium formulation for upper gastrointestinal studies may be suspended over a density range of 60% to 170% w/v at the choice of the user; it is not properly described as a high density barium.

On the question of taste, these barium sulphate preparations for oral administration usually contain sweetening and flavouring agents. Whilst description of one of the latter as a fresh fruit flavour sounds more hopeful than accurate, such additions help to make the drink more acceptable, if not exactly appetizing in nature! A colorant may be added, perhaps to persuade a reluctant recipient that a 'nice taste' is about to be experienced.

Double contrast examinations of the stomach – as we might infer from the term – need the introduction of two radiological contrast agents to the alimentary tract. The technique is used to show fine reticular patterns in the surface of the stomach and depends for success upon what happens to the barium when it flows over the internal surface of the stomach; it must form a thin, smooth coating layer which is free from bubbles and barium precipitates (these mimic small erosions or ulcers). It is to avoid bubble-trapping and precipitation that barium sulphate preparations of high density and low viscosity are especially formulated for these examinations.

Barium sulphate of course is a positive contrast agent (see Barium Preparations in Chapter 4). In a double contrast study it is combined with a gas (carbon dioxide, together with any air swallowed by the patient) to provide negative contrast. The barium is thinly coated over the stomach wall. The swallowing of carbon dioxide then causes distension of the stomach which gives excellent visualization of any small pathological changes which may be present.

Carbon dioxide is administered to the patient orally as an effervescent agent, of which several are available for the purpose, in forms of granules or tablets containing mainly sodium bicarbonate. However, the gas producing agent should be compatible with the barium formulation concerned and it is thus important to use only a combination recommended by the manufacturer of the barium product. In the case of some preparations, an anti-foam agent or bubble breaker has to be added separately to the barium suspension, prior to administration to a patient.

During the investigation, a typical procedure is described in outline below.

(1) To begin the examination, the patient is asked to sit on the X-ray table and takes a prescribed quantity of the gas-producing agent (for instance, the contents of a sachet). With this may be swallowed a small quantity (about 5 ml) of water; or perhaps 10 ml of a special solution (the widely used 'Carbex' contains citric acid, methyl and propylparabens, sodium, saccarine, flavouring and purified water). Depending on the preparation used, 250–700 cm^3 of carbon dioxide are produced.

(2) At this stage the examining radiologist may – or may not – inject the patient with a muscle relaxant. If the small bowel is not to fill with barium and thus possibly overshadow imaged patterns in the stomach, a condition of temporary gastric atony (loss of muscle tone) has often been considered to be essential. To achieve this transiently the patient may be given:

(a) *an anticholinergic drug such as hyoscine butyl bromide ('Buscopan'); or*
(b) *glucagon.*

However, some radiologists may consider drugs unnecessary or may be wary of the several possible side effects, although they may be mild and uncommon (for instance, a patient who has had Buscopan should not drive a car for several hours, as vision may be blurred). Instead a compression technique is employed to keep barium in the stomach. Such a procedure is often quite simple, such as the placing of a firm bolster beneath the abdomen of a prone patient.

(3) The patient takes about 50 ml of the barium sulphate suspension and lies prone on the table, for fluoroscopy and the first of whatever is the standard series of radiographs used in the hospital or by the radiologist concerned.

(4) During the next phase of the examination, the patient drinks – through a straw if he is still recumbent – another 100 ml or so of barium sulphate suspension; the investigation is completed with further survey and filming of the oesophagus and stomach.

Patient management

The careful management by the radiographer of a fluoroscopy session so that it runs well and patients are not waiting for excessive amounts of time is a skill which must be learned. The management of appointment times has already been discussed. There are also ward patients to be scheduled and their transport to the department arranged.

The trolley must be prepared with adequate supplies of cups, contrast agents, other drugs, swabs and so forth.

The room itself must be set up for the procedure; the X-ray couch fitted with handles and footstep; the video-recorder and/or cutfilm camera loaded and readied. Adequate supplies of cassettes must be available and patient identification data prepared. All request forms must be available with previous films and reports.

There may be other people to help with organization, such as nursing staff, but the overall management of the session is the responsibility of the radiographer. Small wonder that many education centres are now formally assessing students on this vital area of their clinical training.

Care of the patient

The barium meal or barium swallow examination will include fluoroscopy and the taking of a number of immediate films. Before the patient leaves the department these are generally processed and checked for quality by either the examining radiologist or a senior radiographer. In many cases this completes the examination and the patient is free to go.

However, it may be that a 'follow-through' series is required; that is, a number of radiographs are taken at later intervals to show the progress of the 'meal' through the small bowel and perhaps the remainder of the alimentary tract. During this procedure the patient may be required to refrain from eating for a further period.

'Accelerators' are often employed to hasten the progress of the contrast agent from the stomach and through the small bowel. The administration of a suitable drug to increase the normal peristaltic rate is advantageous firstly in saving the patient's time and secondly in enabling the radiologist concerned to complete a follow-through examination under fluoroscopic control during the course of a normal morning's session, that is in a total period of about 2 hours.

Glucagon (0.1–0.2 mg given intravenously) has a suitable 'hurrying' effect. Another accelerator which is often used has the proprietary name 'Maxolon' (*metaclopramide monohydrochloride*).

The operation of Maxolon in increasing intestinal peristalsis is on the area of the brain – the hypothalamus – which controls visceral activity; in particular that part which influences the spontaneous movements of the stomach and bowel.

At the end of each patient's fluoroscopic examination the radiographer should ascertain whether or not the procedure is complete and in the latter event know the timing of the further series. This information should be given accurately to the patient, who is entitled also to a word of simple explanation as to what will happen during the remainder of the procedure. It is common to meet with the horrified question, 'Have I got to take any more of that stuff?' – a concern in the circumstances wholly understandable.

Aftercare

Following this examination it is wise to inform patients of the sometimes aggravating effect of barium sulphate on constipation. Barium may be retained in the large bowel of an elderly subject for a very long time (periods of several weeks and even months have been recorded). These people may suffer severe constipation and need attention to their bowel function following a barium meal. Treatment with 50% lactulose ('Duphulac') has been given as a routine after-measure for such patients. Duphulac is a syrup and 5–10 ml may be taken two or three times a day.

Barium sulphate is insoluble and unabsorbable. One of the functions of the colon is to absorb fluid and in the large bowel the barium sulphate mixture becomes denser, solid rather than liquid in character (Howard, 1992). There is a risk that a patient who has a partial intestinal obstruction and to whom a barium meal is given may afterwards become completely obstructed and require immediate surgery. Such patients – if radiological examination of the gastrointestinal tract is necessary – may be given Gastrografin, which is a water-soluble contrast agent and safely excreted by the kidneys.

The other category of patients to whom barium sulphate should not be heedlessly administered by mouth are those suspected of having a gastric leak. This may be from a perforated peptic ulcer or occur because certain joins made during surgery on the stomach break down post-operatively. In either case barium finds its way into the peritoneal cavity and may be difficult to remove by suction or other mechanical means which are the only methods possible. For these patients, too, a Gastrografin meal may be preferable procedure.

Barium enema

Introduction

During a barium enema the large bowel is examined fluoroscopically and radiographs are taken while a suitable barium sulphate mixture is allowed to fill the bowel per rectum. The physical principles of the procedure are identical with those applying to the X-ray examination of other parts of the alimentary tract: a radiopaque fluid is used to fill a body cavity which – if the information obtained is to be diagnostically reliable – must in theory be empty. Ideal preparation of the patient has been achieved when the selected cavity in fact *is* empty.

Preparation of the patient

Allusion has been made earlier to the difficulties inherent in preparing patients for abdominal X-ray examination. When the radiological investigation is to be specifically of the large bowel by barium enema the aim can be simply stated – the colon should be free of all faeces at the time of the examination. Given sufficient care this condition can be achieved; yet a number of patients attending for barium enema have not been sufficiently prepared, for one reason or another.

During the 48 hours prior to examination the patient should take at least 4 pints of fluid and should maintain a low residue diet: eggs, fish, chicken, rusks or crispbread, butter, fruit, milk. It may be wise to omit the previous evening meal but take breakfast, when the X-ray examination is to occur in the morning; and omit breakfast but take a light lunch if the appointment is for the afternoon.

From the evening before the examination, any 'meal' taken should be limited to fluids; clear soups, black coffee or tea – with sugar if desired but not with milk or cream – and fruit drinks suggest themselves: a jelly if it did not contain fruit would be permissible.

Measures – apart from diet – for clearance of the large bowel vary in practice, since there is no definitive procedure which ensures success; and no standard patient of course. As also indicated earlier, the practice of giving washout enemas as preparation has now ceased. The alternative is to use an effective aperient. An example available in the United Kingdom is *X-Prep*, which is a standardized extract of senna fruit. It is presented in individual bottles containing one adult dose (71 ml). In such a form the aperient may easily be handed to an outpatient – or even sent in a pack through the post – and is convenient to take; which the patient should do during the day before the examination between 10 AM and 2 PM.

The 'normal' adult dose of *X-Prep* is prescribed from a formula which allows 1 ml of the extract to be given per kilogram of body weight. Consequently we must be cautious when an adult patient is seen to be thin and frail. A radiographer who is in any doubt of the correct dosage for an individual should seek advice from the referring doctor, a radiologist or pharmacist. All patients should be warned that the drug is likely to produce a strong bowel action and that some spasm or colic may be experienced (Howard, 1992).

Such preparation by means of suitable aperients can effect a satisfactory clearance of the large bowel in most instances. However, aperients are contra-indicated when:

(1) The patient has a colostomy;
(2) There is a history of prolonged diarrhoea;
(3) The patient suffers from Hirchsprung's disease (megacolon).

It should be noted that there are some classes of patients who generally should not be prepared prior to barium examination. These are cases of ulcerative colitis, or of megacolon, or of an acute intussusception.

Preparation and management of the examination

The enema solution
For a barium enema, the solution is more dilute for injection per rectum than when it is to be taken by mouth.

For 'meals', the usual concentrations lie between 3 and 5 g barium sulphate per millilitre of water. For enemas the required concentration is about 1 g barium sulphate per millilitre of water when a double-contrast technique is employed.

There are good reasons for these differences.

(1) During administration per rectum, a thin solution fills the bowel more readily.

(2) If the opacity of the injected solution is high, the mingling images of loops of bowel which overlie each other may be difficult to recognize separately; information may be lost when superimposed opacified loops cannot be visualized 'through' each other.

The employed dilution and the preparation of a barium enema vary with radiological practice; and to some extent with whether or not a pre-filled enema kit is the presentation in question. These kits are used in many X-ray departments. Typically each consists mainly of a plastic bag, measuring approximately 40 cm × 20 cm and already containing a quantity of dry powdered barium sulphate, prepared after the manufacturer's particular formulation. The amount is approximately 500 g barium sulphate but quantities vary and students should look at those stated on any pack in use in their departments. In the upper part of the bag is a snap-closure which allows water to be introduced when the kit is to be used. Finger holes on the upper edge of the bag – and sometimes on both upper and lower edges – permit its suspension during the course of the examination, either by hand or supported by a drip-stand. From the lower part of the bag is brought a length of tubing (about 170 cm) which is closed at its proximal end by a small plastic ball. To this tubing the operator can attach a little ratchet clamp included in the kit; and to the free end of the tubing an appropriate rectal catheter can be fitted.

Preparation of the enema is made as follows.

(1) Fit the ratchet clamp and close the tubing by means of it.

(2) Measure a quantity of warm water (40°C) and add this to the contents of the bag through the snap seal.

At this stage it is necessary of course to know what the required quantity of water is. It affects the 'density' of the enema solution (barium sulphate suspension) expressed as the percentage weight/volume (see Percentage Solutions in Chapter 3). For example, when 2000 ml water are added to a bag containing 400 g barium sulphate, the resultant solution has a density of 20% w/v. A radiologist usually will issue specific instructions for the preparation of a barium enema. In a department where several radiologists work a list may be maintained in the barium preparation room showing the mixture which each requires for enemas; but general guidance can be obtained from manufacturers' data.

(3) Ensure that the snap-seal on the bag is firmly closed.

(4) Hold the bag by the finger holes and shake vigorously for 20 seconds.

(5) Repeat the shaking manoeuvre immediately before use.

(6) 'Pop' the ball from the bag-tube junction with pressure from your

thumb and forefinger (the ball simply floats then on the surface of the barium sulphate suspension). Release of the ball permits the enema to flow from the bag and through the tubing, under control from the ratchet clamp.

(7) Attach the rectal catheter.

(8) The kit is now ready for administration of the enema.

The usual temperature for a barium enema – and indeed others – approximates to normal body heat (37°C; 98°F). To inject a hot solution per rectum is obviously dangerous, and in no circumstances should a warm enema be administered to a patient without a careful check of its temperature being made immediately beforehand. If a warm solution is prepared and has to stand for some while before being used, it is customary to make arrangements to maintain its temperature: for instance, the container may be partly immersed in a bowl of hot water which is frequently renewed.

It is often stated that it is equally undesirable to inject per rectum any solution which is appreciably below blood heat, on the ground that discomfort at least will be caused and in some instances even shock. However, in relation to barium enemata there is some justification for giving the barium at refrigerated temperatures.

The reason for this is that warm solutions produce greater activity of the bowel mucosa, resulting in increased secretion of mucus which may impair its visualization radiographically. When the barium enema can be given chilled, finer detail in the mucosal pattern of the bowel is seen. In regard to the possible effects of low temperature, the patient in many instances seems almost unaware that the solution *is* cold and no unfavourable outcome has been reported – even a literal one in the quick return of the offending mixture.

In some cases, in addition to barium sulphate and water, the enema may contain a bowel evacuant. The presence of an activator assists in the subsequent evacuation of the enema and leads to the remnant barium sulphate appearing as a fine coating over the bowel mucosa, a circumstance of marked diagnostic value when taking the post-evacuation radiographs.

The rectal catheter

For the administration of barium enemata, several devices have been described and are in general use. The simplest is a plain rectal tube of flexible construction, which can very easily be inserted through the anal orifice to a distance of about 7–10 cm. Its major disadvantage is that as it is easy to insert it is equally easy to extrude.

During the fluoroscopic and radiographic examinations the patient will be required to change considerably his position on the X-ray table. Even if a close surveillance of the catheter is made during these manoeuvres, experience shows that it is quite likely to escape from the rectum. These considerations make the administration of a barium enema rather different from enemata of other types and in view of them special varieties of catheter are available.

A typical barium catheter is seen in the upper part of Fig. 6.1. It is made of a firm but fairly flexible plastic material. Flexibility in use is extremely important: an instrument which is rigid would increase the risk of perforating the rectal wall during insertion. The olive-shaped tip of the barium catheter has end-and side-holes and is designed for ease of introduction and to discourage its expulsion: the internal sphincter muscle in the anal canal may grip the 'neck' of the catheter proximally to its expanded head.

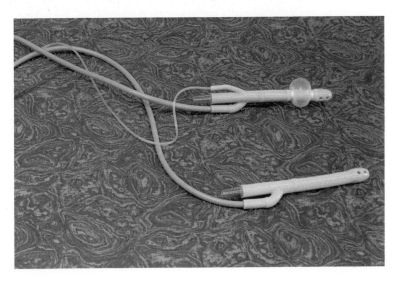

Fig. 6.1 Barium catheters for double contrast studies, an airway being incorporated in each catheter. *Above:* a self-retaining balloon catheter. *Below:* a plain catheter without self-retaining device.

A self-retaining catheter, one example of which is seen in the lower part of Fig. 6.1, is similar in principle to one generally called a Foley catheter. Near its distal end, the catheter is encircled by a small balloon, capable of inflation by means of a separate narrow tube. The catheter is inserted through the anus until the balloon lies completely within the rectum, behind the internal sphincter muscle. Expansion of the balloon by means of a syringe prevents the catheter from passing back through the internal sphincter unless the patient is deliberately attempting to expel it. On completion of the examination, deflation of the balloon allows the catheter to be as easily withdrawn as it was easily inserted.

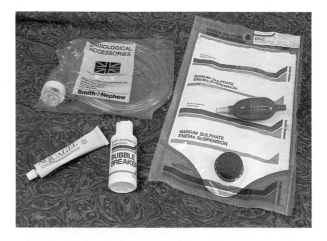

Fig. 6.2 A disposable kit for the barium enema examination which includes, (*left*) lubricant, (*centre*) bubble dispersant, (*right* – on top of enema bag) hand pump for insertion of air.

Either style of catheter may carry an integral airway, a narrow tube entering the catheter at one side to allow the introduction of air during double-contrast studies of the bowel.

All these catheters are usually considered disposable.

For administration of the enema, the bag conveniently may be suspended from its upper edge by means of a dripstand. It is sometimes recommended that during this process the filler cap should be left open since normal air pressure is then maintained, faster delivery ensured and the flow of the enema more precisely controlled.

Introduction of the rectal catheter
When the rectal catheter is ready to be introduced the patient is asked to lie on their left side on the table and to flex the knees towards the chest. The patient is covered with a sheet so that only the area of the buttocks is exposed.

The radiographer puts on gloves and lubricates the end of the rectal catheter with '*KY jelly*' or equivalent (Fig. 6.2). The patient is informed that the tube is about to be inserted and is asked to exhale. The right buttocks should be gently lifted with the heel of your hand to expose the anus. The catheter tip is gently inserted approximately 7.5 cm towards the umbilicus (see Fig. 6.3). The tube must **never** be inserted forcefully as this may cause rupture of the mucous membranes (Torres, 1989).

The use of the left lateral position for insertion follows the natural anatomy of the sigmoid colon (Pritchard & Mallett, 1992).

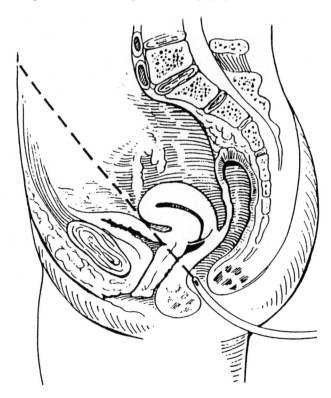

Fig. 6.3 Insertion of a rectal catheter. The dotted line shows the direction of insertion of the tube which should be towards the umbilicus and inserted approximately 7.5 cm. *(Reproduced by courtesy of J.B. Lippincott Co, USA.)*

When the tip is inserted it should be initially held in place with the hand and the fluid allowed to run in slowly.

When a retaining catheter is used the inflatable cuff should only be inflated by a radiologist owing to the dangers of perforation with this type of catheter (Chapman & Nakielny, 1993).

When it is desired to obtain evacuation of the enema, the bag – with its filler cap safely closed – is removed from the stand and simply lowered to a position below the level of the X-ray table when the barium mixture should flow back into it. Evacuation may thus take place under maintained fluoroscopic control and the post-evacuation films can be easily and expeditiously exposed. When the procedure is completed the enema bag is clipped off and the whole arrangement discarded as it is. It is very important that at no stage in the administration of the enema should the container be raised to a great height above the table. To do this is directly to increase the pressure at which the enema is given. Such pressure can be dangerous should the bowel wall be thinned and delicate, as it is in the presence of ulcerative colitis; and in any case high pressure makes retention of the enema difficult and unlikely.

One or two air-bulb syringes (Fig. 6.2) of the type known as a Higginson's syringe will be required in the case of a double-contrast examination, which entails the insufflation of air to the large bowel, after partial evacuation of the barium enema. Alternatively, air may be administered using the enema bag itself as a 'pump'.

An enema ring or retainer (Fig. 6.4) is a useful accessory since it restricts the spread of a flood of barium in the event of the patient's being unable to retain the enema. It consists of a small circular plastic sheet, attached to the periphery of which is an inflatable ring – placed beneath the patient's buttocks when the device is in use. The arrangement rather resembles a miniature of those inflatable paddling pools obtainable as garden toys for children. Should leakage of the enema occur, it is contained within the ring and its disposal is subsequently easy and complete, particularly if a paper towel has been placed in the ring to receive it. The device is quite radiolucent and does not seriously interfere with fluoroscopic or radiographic detail. Since it offers rather a cold surface to the patient's skin, the enema ring may be made more comfortable by the insertion of a circle of gauze, cellulose wadding or a paper towel. This has another advantage: it keeps the ring 'clean' for the next patient.

Care of the patient

While the patient is being made ready for barium enema examination, it is kind to give some explanation of what is about to happen. Recent articles

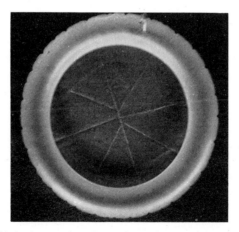

Fig. 6.4 A disposable barium retainer. It may be used more than once if it is covered with a paper towel and the patient retains the enema. *(Reproduced by courtesy of Med-Co Hospital Supplies Ltd.)*

have commented critically on the adequacy of such explanations (Ferguson, 1988; Howard, 1992).

Often the examining radiologist includes an explanation in discussing with the patient their medical history; but not all are equally careful in this respect. Radiographers should recognize their own obligations in the matter and make sure that the patient fully understands:

(1) That they will receive an enema, and what the examination entails;
(2) That they will lie on a hard table and that it may move during the procedure;
(3) That they will be asked to move into different positions while retaining the enema solution.

As a preliminary we should comfort the patient about retention of the enema which is necessary for a short period. A positive outlook should be encouraged by an explanation that the enema mixture is not irritant to the bowel and that it is not designed or intended to produce evacuation; it may also be useful to refer to the feature of fluoroscopy which allows us 'to see exactly what is happening inside' and thus prevent discomfort.

However, inevitably there are some patients who prove unable to retain the enema with success, particularly perhaps the elderly in whom the anal sphincter may have become lax. When this happens, almost all experience feelings of distress and even shame, residual memories of childhood's guilt over such lapses.

We have a responsibility here to reassure the patient that they are neither a nuisance nor the cause of censure. We should tell them with a smile how well accustomed we are to this minor difficulty, which is a recognized and may be a frequent feature of this examination. Mopping-up operations should be conducted expeditiously and without comment, and the patient gently encouraged to do their best to allow the examination to continue. Soothing techniques and the use of therapeutic touch to ease anxiety during the examination have been researched and advocated by DeCann (1990) and DeCann & Hegarty (1993).

In its simplest form a barium enema examination has two fluoroscopic phases.

(1) Under visual observation and control, the large bowel is filled with the contrast enema. During this phase radiographs are obtained at the radiologist's discretion in order to record observed appearances and to assist diagnosis.
(2) Further fluoroscopy follows evacuation of the enema and again radio-graphs are obtained; when appropriate these post-evacuation films may include exposures made with the over-table X-ray tube.

It is now correct radiological practice to complement the second phase of the examination with an air study (double contrast enema): that is, air is introduced per rectum, which will distend the lumen and project the mucosa of the bowel in a relief pattern. The detection of any small polyp thus becomes more likely; this may be an important finding for a patient, since untreated polyps have a significant ultimate tendency towards malignant change.

Whilst it is now very common, the use of double contrast is not invariable practice, since the procedure has two recognizable disadvantages:

(1) It is uncomfortable, the majority of patients finding air insufflation more distressing than the introduction of the original barium enema;
(2) It prolongs the investigation; this inevitably increases the fret for a patient and may reduce the number of patients who can be examined during the course of any single session.

Consequently experienced radiologists may be found to select in some circumstances the simpler procedure; for example, in the case of a patient who is very old and frail or whose clinical history is without relevance.

On the point of the length of time needed for a barium enema examination, the implications for a double-contrast technique should be kept in mind when making appointments and advising a patient of the period likely to be required. It is probably better to overestimate than to give the impression that the examination can be concluded within a few minutes (Ferguson, 1988).

The evacuatory stage of the enema is worth attention for reasons of patient-care. During the examination a sufficiently effective evacuation can be obtained if the rectal catheter *in situ* and the enema bag are used as a siphon, the enema bag simply being lowered to the floor to obtain a down-flow. However, the situation should not then be deemed to be a completed act. A radiographer who considers it so behaves unwisely.

Following a barium enema, no patient should be allowed to dress and leave the department without *first* going to the lavatory. In some cases, as a result of the siphoning process, little discomfort is felt and the patient may firmly believe that there is no immediate need to evacuate further. Such patients depart eagerly to get dressed, glad to put on their clothes and assume again responsibility for themselves. If the radiographer has failed to give warning and has allowed this situation to occur, it has been known that the hospital was afterwards obliged to settle an account for the cost of cleaning a suit.

Elderly patients, or those in a weakened condition, should not be dispatched to the lavatory and left unattended for any length of time. In a few instances the patient may become suddenly shocked and faint. It is far better that we should many times give supervision more often than is necessary to the comparatively fit, than that we should once fail to be near at hand when the patient's need was real.

The patient with a colostomy

A colostomy is a surgical procedure in which the colon is opened on to the surface of the abdomen. This is done so as to provide an artificial outlet for the faecal contents of the colon, the patient's bowel motions being discharged through this opening and not through the anus from the rectum in the normal way. Colostomy is undertaken for two main reasons:

(1) To construct a permanent 'artificial anus' when the rectum is to be surgically removed because it is diseased;
(2) To construct a temporary diversion route for the faecal contents when it is thought advisable for the distal part of the colon not to function for a time.

So a temporary colostomy may be established as part of a treatment plan when the distal colon is obstructed or inflamed or perforated or is to be the subject of difficult surgery.

A permanent colostomy is what is known as a terminal or end colostomy. Distal to the colostomy there is no bowel remaining, the colostomy opening being the end of the line (if we make an analogy with the railway track). The rectum is surgically removed and the sigmoid colon is brought out as a colostomy opening on the anterior abdominal wall; a favoured site is the left iliac fossa. In the case of a temporary arrangement planned to stop the distal colon functioning, a loop of transverse colon is used to construct the colostomy. The siting of a transverse colostomy of this kind is often to the right of the midline in the upper quadrant of the abdomen (that is, between the umbilicus and the lower costal margin). In this type of colostomy there is bowel remaining distal to the abdominal opening and usually there is still an anal orifice at the extreme distal end of the bowel.

Radiographers are confronted with either type of colostomy in patients coming to the X-ray department. When a patient with a terminal colostomy arrives for a radiological contrast enema, the only possibility for giving it is through the colostomy opening. If the colostomy is temporary there are usually *two* routes of access: via the colostomy or via the anus. Selection of route for a particular examination depends on why it is being made, which part of the colon it is wished to study and whether the anus provides a satisfactory opening (it may be narrowed or obstructed or damaged as a result of a disease process). If the anus is used for entry point when an enema is given to a patient with a colostomy the enema solution of course will shortly appear through the colostomy opening.

In the case of a baby born with an imperforate anus there is no anal opening at all. Temporary colostomy may then be done on the new-born and at a later stage, when the child is bigger and stronger, surgery to construct an anal canal may be planned. The child may be X-rayed at that stage with a view to finding out how much colon there is distal to the colostomy opening. Clearly then the contrast enema must be given into the distal colon through the colostomy opening as there is no other way in.

Temporary colostomy often has a double-barrelled construction in which two entrance points present themselves at the colostomy opening. The two openings are separated by a spur of tissues which has been organized to prevent the faecal contents of the bowel passing over from the one opening to the other. Of the two openings, the one further to the patient's right is the active one through which the bowel discharges its contents in its action. A catheter inserted in this opening can be used to fill with contrast agent that part of the colon which is proximal to the colostomy. The other opening (the one further to the patient's left) leads to the inactive remaining bowel. If a catheter is inserted here the distal part of the colon is filled. When an enema is given to a patient with a colostomy, the solution must be delivered at a low pressure and the container must not be raised too high.

By whatever route an enema is injected, the patient has no voluntary control over evacuation through a colostomy. So it is a waste of effort for us to tell them that they must try to retain the enema as if we were instructing a patient whose evacuation arrangements were normal. This patient has no sphincters for his colostomy for there are no muscles of this type around the opening. Radiographers dealing with colostomy patients must be prepared for various approaches in regard to giving the enema; lack of control of evacuation through a colostomy is, however, a constant feature to be understood.

Management of a colostomy

The patient with a permanent colostomy has to learn to live with a new arrangement for defecation. The patient will receive help and advice for this while in hospital for the operation and, as time goes by, will learn management of the colostomy. As we have seen, the patient is never able to *control* it but the bowel adjusts itself. The colostomy actions become less frequent than in the immediate post-operative period and eventually the patient may find that the colostomy behaves in a predictable way, acting at regular times in the day (such as after a main meal) perhaps only once, perhaps twice or more.

It is easy to see that the patient will manage best when the motions are firm, are not too frequent and are predictable. Aid in achieving this stage of affairs can be found by attention to diet and if necessary by the use of certain medicines.

Colostomy appliances

Various appliances are available for management of a colostomy. The commonest practice now is for the patient to wear a disposable plastic bag over the opening. When the colostomy functions, the results are held securely in the bag until the patient can attend to it, dispose of the used bag and fit another. Patients with colostomies will be found to carry with them spare plastic bags and cleaning materials to enable them to make changes while away from home. It is not a bad idea for the X-ray department to include among its stores some spare colostomy bags.

The plastic bags which are used come in two main types: (1) those which are adherent and stick directly on to the patient's skin around the colostomy; and (2) those which are non-adherent and are held on to the patient over the opening by some type of belt or corset. The non-adherent type of bag attaches to a rigid or semi-rigid plastic ring or flange which fits over the colostomy opening and is kept in position by the colostomy belt.

One of the disadvantages of using adherent bags is that the patient's skin may become sore, especially if removal and renewal of the bags must be done two or three times in the course of 24 hours. There is an appliance which avoids both the encumbrance of a belt and the necessity for frequent changing of an adherent bag. This is achieved by means of a rigid plastic flange which has an adhesive square on its back surface. The flange is thereby stuck directly to the skin around the colostomy opening. It can be left in place for two or three days and a new bag is simply fitted to the free rim of the flange as often as is necessary.

A patient with his colostomy so well regulated that he is confident of no action during the day may be found to wear very little in the way of an appliance – perhaps a small dressing of cellulose wadding held in place by a belt of light elasticated fabric.

Small bowel enema

This is an examination which is becoming more common and in certain centres is replacing the barium 'follow-through' as the examination of choice. It is said to give better visualization of the small bowel (Chapman & Nakielny, 1993, p. 60).

A tube is introduced via the pharynx directly into the distal part of the duodenum. Because of this the preparation and patient care for this examination are very similar to that required for endoscopic retrograde cholangiopancreatography (ERCP) and therefore the two examinations will be considered together in Chapter 8 on the biliary system.

References

Chapman, S. & Nakielny, R. (1993) *A Guide to Radiological Procedures*, (pages 60, 68), 3rd Edn., Baillière Tindall, London.

DeCann, R. (1990) Soothing techniques used in barium enema examinations. *Radiography Today*, 56 (639), 18–20.

DeCann, R. & Hegarty, J. (1993) Soothing techniques in radiography – do staff do what they say they do? *Radiography Today*, 59 (676), 13–16.

Ferguson, M. (1988) The person inside the patient. *Nursing Times*, 84 (51), 40.

Howard, A. (1992) An enema hath done this. *Radiography Today*, 58 (663), 35.

Pritchard, A.P. & Mallett, J. (1992) *Manual of Clinical Nursing Procedures*, (page 96), 3rd Edn., Blackwell Science, Oxford.

Torres, L.S. (1989) *Basic Medical Techniques and Patient Care for Radiologic Technologists*, (pages 106–7), 3rd Edn., JB Lippincott Company, Philadelphia.

Chapter 7
The Renal Tract

Plain radiographs of the renal tract are taken but they do not constitute the most useful procedure unless there are present known radiopaque calculi, the progress of which it is desired to assess. A plain film of the abdomen will generally indicate the size, shape, and position of each kidney but a proportion of all urinary stones are translucent to X-rays; their degree of opacity depends entirely on the salts of which they are composed. Those containing a high content of calcium carbonate are in fact markedly radio-paque and show well on a plain radiograph.

However, other calcium salts such as calcium oxylate and calcium phosphate are commonly present. Some urinary calculi may prove wholly radioparent and incapable of plain radiographic demonstration against the tissues which normally surround them. In this case a radiological report which states that 'There is no evidence of a renal calculus', or that 'No abnormality is detected', cannot be taken to mean that no stone is present, or that all is necessarily well with this patient. Such information is clearly of limited value.

These considerations usually make it preferable to undertake X-ray investigations of the renal tract which incorporate the introduction of a contrast medium and from which the presence and site of a radioparent stone may be inferred by its effect on the functioning and the appearance of the system. Since a plain 'scout' film is always taken at the beginning of these special investigations, any radiopaque stones will be identified from this; the subsequent procedure can further assist in their localization, should there be any doubt of the shadows being due to the presence of calcified mesenteric glands. In many cases, ultrasound is now the investigation of first choice.

Intravenous urography

Intravenous urography is the most frequently performed of the special investigations relating to the urinary tract. It has several advantages.

(1) It is a simple procedure for the patient which does not involve the passing of instruments or the induction of anaesthesia.

(2) It gives information on the efficacy of renal function and is the only X-ray examination to do this.
(3) Providing there is adequate function of the kidneys, satisfactory detail of the structure of the renal system can be obtained which may lead to the diagnosis of other lesions than calculi; for example renal tuberculosis.

The procedure of intravenous urography (sometimes termed *excretion urography, descending urography or IVP* for intravenous pyelography) implies the injection into a vein – usually in the antecubital fossa at the elbow – of a suitable contrast agent which is rapidly excreted by the kidneys. It will normally appear in the renal tract in a matter of minutes and delineate the whole renal system in a series of radiographs taken at short intervals following injection.

Preparation of the patient

When making the appointment the patient should be warned that the examination is likely to occupy approximately an hour. It is questionable whether or not he should be told also that he will be given a simple injection of a 'dye' which will assist in obtaining better X-ray films. Many people have a disproportionate dislike of injections. They view this procedure with an irrational nervousness which can scarcely be related to the momentary and usually trivial pain of the needle's insertion: indeed such sufferers often accept stoically physical pangs far more severe.

It is most important that when the patient *is* told of the coming injection, they should receive the additional information that it should not affect them in any way.

Physical preparation of the patient often consists of the form of general abdominal preparation current in the department (Chapter 5) together with some possible restriction of the patient's intake of fluid. The reason for this is to obtain concentration of the contrast medium in the renal pelves and therefore visualization of radiographic detail. If the patient has taken much to drink immediately prior to intravenous urography this will of course be reflected in the renal drainage system by increased urinary excretion. Dilution of the radiopaque agent with urine may lead to reduced contrast and consequently loss of perception of radiographic detail in the pyelogram.

The extent of the restriction actually imposed on the patient will vary between departments, depending on the wishes of the radiologist in charge. A severe regimen of hydration may defeat its own ends as in these circumstances renal function may be much reduced. A specific optimum period of dehydration has not been established and, provided that the contrast agent can be given in an adequate amount, a satisfactory result will be obtained in a patient who has received no special preparation at all. For this reason, many departments have now abandoned the practice. Students should inquire what is current in their own department (Maclennan, 1992).

Dehydration should not be applied to anyone who is in renal failure or suffering from multiple myeloma.

For the purpose again of preventing dilution of the contrast agent, it is of considerable importance that the bladder should be empty when intravenous urography is performed. If this is not so, radiographic visualization will be impaired when the medium enters the bladder and its detail may never be adequately demonstrated. Attention should be paid to this when the patient is making ready for the examination: they should be requested to visit the lavatory immediately before undressing.

When intravenous urography is performed as an emergency procedure no long-term preparation of the patient is possible and the emptying of the bladder is the only essential preliminary.

A child or infant who is to have an intravenous urogram should not be prepared with a laxative and must not be subjected to a lengthy period of dehydration.

Preparation of the injection

When any hypodermic injection is given the rules of asepsis must be strictly observed. Infection can very easily follow if practice is allowed to become lax in this respect. The technique of intravenous urography is simple. It is at the same time so frequently performed in many departments as to become a commonplace of every day's work: perhaps there is some danger that its risks – if it receives only a careless attention – may be overlooked or disregarded. We have all of us a real responsibility in this respect and should maintain continuous vigilance in the preparing and handling of any sterile equipment.

In current practice it is likely that the sterile items for this procedure are disposable and prepacked. A radiographer preparing the trolley might obtain these commodities from a stock in the department's clean utility room, to the shelves of which they would have come from the hospital's central sterile supply area. The packages should be placed in an orderly arrangement on the trolley's top shelf, but none is opened until the injection is about to be administered.

Trolley setting – sterile

- Syringes, usually 50 ml (Fig. 7.1).
- One or two 10 cm (5 inches) cannulae for drawing up contrast agent.
- One or two 'butterfly' needles.
- Needles in sizes appropriate to the syringes.

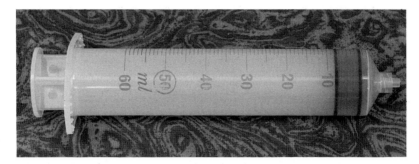

Fig. 7.1 Pre-sterilized disposable syringe for intravenous administration of a contrast agent (see also Figures 3.1 and 3.2).

- Injection swabs ('Sterets') for skin cleansing. These prepared swabs are already saturated with 70% isopropyl alcohol and each is presented in an individual pack.

Trolley-setting – non sterile

- Phials of the contrast agent to be used; for example 'Conray 420' in a 50 ml bottle.
- A bowl containing cotton wool swabs. These will be used to apply finger pressure to the injection site, so as to limit bleeding when a needle is withdrawn from a vein.
- A few small 'plaster' dressings of a familiar first-aid type, for subsequent application to the injection site.
- A roll of narrow adhesive tape, for securing the butterfly needle, if this is used.
- A pair of scissors.
- A tourniquet.
- A small sandbag or padded board for support of the arm.
- A receiver in case of vomiting.

The injection of a urographic contrast agent is a task for the medically qualified; it should be undertaken only by a radiologist or other doctor. In some hospitals, however, radiographers are now receiving special training to carry out injections themselves. This is an example of *role extension*. The usual role, however, is to assist in the procedure, and, in doing this, there are some points which must be noticed by the radiographer.

(1) Whilst it is not necessary to 'scrub', the hands should be newly washed and clean.
(2) The syringe should be grasped by the barrel to remove it from its sealed paper pack and should not be handled unnecessarily often; in particular the nozzle should be kept away from any non-sterile surface.

(3) The warning above applies equally to the cannula of both extremities of which special care should be taken, first whilst removing its covering and secondly whilst fitting the cannula to the syringe nozzle.

(4) When the phial of contrast agent is opened the mouth of the bottle must not be touched with the fingers or otherwise contaminated. The contents of the phial must be examined to see that they are in good condition, and that the expiry date has not been exceeded.

(5) During filling of the syringe, the end of the cannula should be plunged directly into the fluid, without touching any external part of the bottle.

(6) The empty bottle should be retained on the trolley until conclusion of the X-ray examination.

It is *most important* that the agent to be injected should be checked at every stage of the procedure – when the trolley is prepared and again when the agent is taken into the syringe. The radiographer must check it and must see that the doctor also checks it *before* giving the injection. From time to time disasters occur in hospital because a patient has been injected with the wrong substance; failure to check constantly and efficiently allows these things to occur.

When the doctor comes to give the injection, the tourniquet should be put round the patient's arm sufficiently far above the elbow to leave the bend of the elbow well clear for the injection site. The tourniquet is tightened enough to distend the veins, and it will assist in this if the patient can help by opening and closing his fist several times.

If the agent to be injected is contained in a single dose ampoule, this will be opened by the radiographer when the doctor is ready. The ampoule neck is marked with a file. The ampoule should be broken at the filed neck, being held for this purpose in a piece of sterile gauze. The radiographer then holds the ampoule while the doctor draws the contents into the syringe.

The radiographer should check the name on the label and see that the doctor also checks it. As has been indicated, the importance of this can hardly be over-emphasized.

Cleansing of the patient's skin at the injection site may be done by the doctor just before giving the injection. The radiographer will steady the patient's arm, which should rest on a small sandbag or firm pad, and will observe and reassure the patient. When the needle is in the vein, the doctor will check that it is so by drawing blood back into the syringe before proceeding with the injection. At this point, when the blood is seen in the syringe, the radiographer or the doctor will release the tourniquet.

The emergency tray

The student will know from Chapter 3 that many radiological contrast agents contain iodine and that some individuals are sensitive to this element.

Such people may rapidly develop unpleasant and possibly dangerous reactions, if they have to take any substance containing iodine, particularly – and this is a significant point – if it is introduced directly into the blood-stream by way of an artery or vein. In any X-ray room where such procedures are undertaken there should be permanently available an emergency tray and equipment for the administration of restorative drugs and other measures. The need for this equipment may be prevented by the use of non-ionic contrast agents (e.g. *omnipaque*) in patients who have a known history of allergy (see Adverse Reactions, below).

Care of the patient

During the preliminaries for intravenous urography some explanation of the procedure should be given to the patient. Our patient not only may be seeing for the first time the ritual of preparation for intravenous injection, but is well aware that they will be at the receiving end of a syringe which looks at first glimpse more suitable in size to a horse. A little sympathetic reassurance may be comforting beyond our knowledge.

It should be mentioned that apart from the needle's prick little else will be felt from the injection. Certainly in skilled hands and providing the needle is sharp – literally and figuratively, this is a very important point – many patients may be hardly aware that the injection has been given, perhaps particularly those who are nervous beforehand.

It is a mistake to attempt to quiet an alarmed child by saying 'It will not hurt'. Within a very short time this is manifestly proved an untruth and that child will not readily trust us again. We can fairly say that 'it will hurt a little', but that if they are brave this part will be over quickly and that all we have to do then is to take a few pictures.

As far as possible all preparations for the injection and the instruments to be used should be kept out of sight of the child, who should be spoken to cheerfully and encouraged to look away while the injection is made.

Following it the patient should not be left alone until at least 15 or 20 minutes have elapsed. Here again it is worth bearing in mind that our attitude may easily become conditioned by the familiarity and general safety of the procedure. If the patient does experience adverse effects from the contrast agent, they may appear at any subsequent time but most probably they will occur during this quarter of an hour.

It is true of course that such an emergency is a rarity. It may not happen within the working experience of any one radiographer, and because of this we find ourselves believing that it will not happen at all. Usually we are right. Many times we may leave the patient for a few moments but in these circumstances we can never do so in safety. The risk remains that on some occasion on returning to the room we shall find the patient extremely ill; it is no overstatement that in this event a few minutes' earlier attention could have altered the balance between death and life.

Adverse reactions

The reactions which may occur are categorized as arising from:

(1) Toxic effects of the injected chemical;
(2) Osmolar effects;
(3) Allergic effects.

The first two of these have been briefly considered (see Chapter 3 under the heading Iodine Preparations). The last are idiosyncratic reactions and when true allergy occurs it is independent of the dose given.

Some workers have produced evidence which suggests that allergic-type reactions to radiological contrast agents may not be characterized by the production of antibodies – the antigen/antibody mechanism – and cannot correctly be ascribed to an allergy in the patient. Be these reservations as they may, some patients react to the injection of a radiological contrast agent with symptoms which are recognized manifestations of allergy.

Allergy is an altered reaction of the tissues of some individuals on exposure to substances which in similar quantities are innocuous to most people. More simply we can say that the person concerned has a peculiar sensitivity to the substance.

An agent which produces allergy is known as an *allergen* or *antigen*. Almost any substance is capable of exciting a reaction of this kind: it may be a food such as fish or strawberries; it may be an inhalant such as the pollen of some plants or chemical fumes; it may be a drug.

It is unusual for an allergic subject to be sensitive to only one allergen. Multiple sensitivities are the rule. A person known to be sensitive to other antigens may be at particular risk when a radiological contrast agent is introduced to the blood stream.

For this reason, before embarking on a procedure which requires direct injection of one of the organic iodine compounds into a blood vessel, the examining radiologist should take a careful history from the patient to establish that he is not an allergic subject; the patient may be asked, for example, whether he has ever suffered from hay fever or asthma since each of these conditions is a manifestation of allergy. A specific enquiry should be made as to whether he has ever been told tht he is allergic to anything. Typical of a mild allergic reaction are soreness and running of the eyes and the appearance of an urticarial rash over the body: this may be a faint patchy blush or may be very pronounced, the patient becoming heavily covered with large, red, irritating weals.

In more serious cases bronchospasm can occur, or laryngeal oedema (swelling of the mucous membrane) may be so marked as vitally to impair breathing. If the respiratory disturbance is sufficiently severe, *tracheostomy* may be necessary: this is a means of creating an artificial airway through an incision in the front of the neck, the opening being kept patent for as long as required by the insertion of a tracheostomy tube (see Chapter 9).

To suppress an allergic state the most effective drugs are the corticosteroids which – given intravenously – act in about 30 minutes. Adrenaline may be used for an acute condition as it obtains results much more rapidly (in 2 or 3 minutes). The antihistamine preparations (for example, Phenergan) are more appropriate for preventing a reaction than for treating it.

If a patient has a known history of allergies, a non-ionic (LOCM) contrast agent will be administered.

A particular form of hypersensitivity to an allergen is a condition known as *anaphylaxis*, in which a subject has been sensitized specifically to an allergen by some previous inoculation. When such a patient receives a further injection, for example of a radiological contrast agent during urography, they experience a profound circulatory collapse. Blood pressure falls rapidly and cataclysmically; pulses become undetectable; the patient presents the desperate picture of extreme shock (anaphylactic shock). On some occasions, breathing may stop (respiratory arrest) and cessation of the heart's beat (cardiac arrest) can occur. Every member of the X-ray staff should know what to do in an emergency of this kind. (This is described in detail in the first section of Chapter 17). Anaphylactic shock is a very dangerous, though infrequent, occurrence, of which unhappily no previous indication is received of the subject who may suffer it. As indicated earlier, the use of non-ionic contrast agents in certain categories of patients such as those over a particular age (e.g. 65) will hopefully reduce this incidence even further.

A radiographer, undertaking intravenous urography and attending a patient in the throes of unpleasant after-effects from an injection, of course is more concerned with immediate signs and symptoms, than precisely with causes of the patient's malaise; it is necessary to recognize those reactions of minimal effect, and those which are significant.

Minor reactions are not unusual and include:

(1) Warmth;
(2) Nausea and perhaps vomiting;
(3) Faintness and palpitations;
(4) Arm pain and perhaps headache.

As a rule, these effects pass quickly. Reassurance and comfortable covering of the patient often are all that is required. A nauseated patient should be supplied with a receiver (the provision of which sometimes coincides happily with abatement of the nausea).

Medical attention should be obtained when vomiting or headache is severe or prolonged or when other changes in a patient's condition are observed.

Any reaction suggestive of an allergy must be considered as significant, even when a symptom is mild. Medical help should be sought immediately for any of the following:

(1) Urticaria;
(2) Bronchospasm (the patient is obviously distressed in his breathing;
(3) Laryngeal oedema (there is difficulty in swallowing and breathing);
(4) Anaphylactic shock (Chapman & Nakielny, 1993).

For many patients, urticaria may be the only manifestation of allergy and may be so slight so as to appear not to need treatment; but potentially it is a forerunner of the more dangerous conditions which have been described. Especially may it be of moment for a patient who will have a subsequent contrast agent examination.

Any patient who experiences a marked reaction following urography will naturally remain under close medical observation in the department for a period. Admission to hospital for at least 24 hours may be considered advisable, particularly in the case of an anaphylactic collapse.

Cystography: cysto-urethrography

The lower urinary tract may be visualized by the direct injection of a suitable contrast agent. Cystography implies that the bladder alone is examined. Its usefulness is limited and – in view of the availability of other forms of diagnostic image – it is now virtually off the scene. Wider in application is the complete investigation of both bladder and urethra denoted by the expression *cysto-urethrography*. Cysto-urethrography includes *micturating cystography* (in which the urethra is visualized radiologically during micturition) and *ascending urethrography* (when the male urethra is filled with a contrast agent by means of a distal injection).

The student will find that the radiographic procedures to be followed show a marked variation which is dependent mainly upon the reasons for the investigation and in part on the individual wishes of urologist and radiologist.

The anatomical dissimilarities of the lower urinary tract between the sexes influence the pathology which may occur and necessitate the use of differing techniques when cysto-urethrography is performed.

Because the male urethra is longer and more devious in its course, it is much more readily obstructed than the female: patients suspected of having a urethral stricture and presenting for cysto-urethrography as a rule are male. The same anatomical features make the urethra and bladder of the male more difficult to catheterize and special instruments may be employed for the introduction of a radiological contrast agent to demonstrate the urethra.

In women, incompetence of the internal sphincter muscle surrounding the internal urethral orifice may lead to a condition called stress incontinence: the patient loses control of her bladder during activities – such as coughing or laughing – which raise intraabdominal pressure. Cystography is commonly employed to prove inadequacy of the sphincter in such patients. In this case the important radiographic views are lateral projections of the bladder and urethra exposed when the patient is at rest or straining and during micturition. In women, catheterization is generally a simple job and the special equipment needed for the radiological procedure is primarily the provision of a suitable commode or its equivalent which will allow films to be exposed while the patient passes urine in a customary posture.

Thus, cysto-urethrography cannot satisfactorily be classed as one procedure and is difficult to present to the student alone a single line, in the manner of other diagnostic X-ray examinations which are described in this book. The following paragraphs no more than sketch certain significant features of these investigations. However, it is hoped that they may provide readers with guidance to the techniques practised in their own X-ray departments. In many departments, such examinations are numerous, owing to the prevalence of urinary incontinence as a condition, particularly in an ageing population.

Preparation of the patient

Points to be noted in the preparation of the patient include the following.

(1) Some of these investigations are not usually performed on outpatients. Children or very apprehensive patients may require mild sedation to secure co-operation.

(2) Application of routine radiological abdominal preparation. Shaving of the pubic hair is not usually considered necessary.

(3) Explanation of the procedure and reassurance of the patient.

(4) Emptying of the bladder immediately prior to the examination.

(5) Insertion of the catheter or urethral cannula under strictly sterile conditions. In some instances the patient may come to the X-ray room with a catheter in place.

(6) Withdrawal of residual urine into a suitable receiver. In some cases its measurement may be necessary.

Preparation of the trolley

The trolley should be made ready in sterile and non-sterile sections. The sterility of any instrument or substance introduced to the urethra and bladder is very important, as the lower urinary tract easily becomes infected. The specialized equipment required must vary depending on the examination. However, the following observations may be helpful.

(1) For male urethrography it is usual to employ a special cannula for the introduction of the contrast agent. This instrument may be one which is known as a Knutson's clamp and is depicted in Fig. 7.2. The method of use is perhaps evident from the illustration. The clamp supports both the cannula and the penis, the pillar and the bars of the clamp being adjusted to hold the two in line with each other, once the acorn tip has been placed within the urethral orifice.

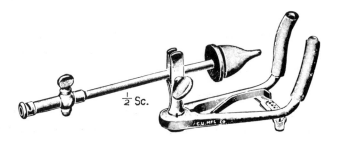

Fig. 7.2 Knutson's clamp and cannula for male urethrography. *(Reproduced by courtesy of the Genito-Urinary Manufacturing Co Ltd.)*

A more elegant and pleasant instrument for the purpose is found in the Malmstrom–Thoren vacuum uterine cannula. The use of a uterine cannula for male urethrography (the ultimate in unisex) may surprise the reader. However, the instrument is readily made suitable by means of annular adaptors of different sizes to fit the glans penis.

The Malmstrom–Thoren equipment consists of:

(a) A hand-operated vacuum pump which need not be sterile for the procedure;
(b) A cannula and its piston;
(c) A number of glass cone-shaped cups of different sizes, with screws and washers;
(d) A variety of rubber acorns.

Items (b), (c) and (d) require to be sterile during the procedure and may be kept ready for use in a suitable sterilizing solution, such as chlorhexidine.

In use the equipment is assembled so that the acorn is withdrawn in the glass cup. An 'O' ring (modified pill-box lid) of suitable size is pressed in position at the distal end of the cup, in which a vacuum will be produced by the operation of the attached pump. When the acorn is introduced to the urethral orifice and the 'O' ring applied to the glans penis, vacuum pressure (of about 0.3–0.4 kg/cm^2) almost at once holds the cannula and the tissues painlessly and retentively together. The instrumentation is relatively comfortable for the patient and virtually all leakage of the contrast agent is prevented; if a little reflux should occur it is not significant radiologically, as it is collected in the cup and does not interfere with radiographic appearances.

Although here described with reference to male urethrography, the technique is equally satisfactory for female patients. The vacuum cup and its 'O' ring create a seal with the female periurethral tissues as effectively as with the glans penis.

(2) In the absence of such special equipments as have been described, self-retaining balloon catheters or simple soft catheters of suitable sizes will be needed. In examination for stress incontinence, a fine radiopaque catheter may be used as it assists delineation of urethro-vesical relationships, which are significant for diagnosis.

(3) In the case of male patients a local anaesthetic may be considered necessary. A suitable one is 2% xylocaine antiseptic gel, of which 3–4 ml are introduced through the urinary meatus by means of the catheter or cannula in place.

(4) The radiological contrast agents in general use for cysto-urethrography are water-soluble, organic iodine compounds. Up to 20 ml may be injected under fluoroscope observation and radiographs to the examining radiologist's choice are exposed at intervals by means of the serial changer associated with the fluoroscopic table.

(5) Radiographs exposed during micturition are often essential to cysto-urethrography. They require obviously the provision of an appropriate urinary receiver. The nature of this and the way in which it is used must depend on the examination in question.

For example, a man may find urination difficult or impossible when he is recumbent: consequently thought should be given to arrangements which will permit the exposures during micturition to be made whilst the patient is upright, if he is physically capable of standing.

During examinations for female stress incontinence, a disposable bed-pan (which has the virtue of radiolucency), placed on a wooden stool (or one of some other radiulucent material), is a simple contrivance which allows a patient to micturate in a normal manner while lateral radiographs are taken by means of a vertical bucky or cassette holder.

Care of the patient

Care of the patient will follow general principles of comfort and reassurance during these rather exacting procedures. Many, even adult patients, may have difficulty in initiating micturition to order. The provision of reasonable privacy is a significant factor which will mean much to the sensitive patient, and may indeed mark the difference between a successful and an unsatisfactory examination. To this end, the coming and going through the X-ray room of staff not directly concerned in the procedure are to be avoided and the number of people present should, whenever possible, not be more than is necessary to its proper conduct. Students attending for instructional purposes should be confined to a small group.

In regard to young children, difficulty in obtaining the radiographs during micturition may be pronounced, owing to the child's reluctance or inability to initiate the act. External stimuli can be utilized. The suggestive effect of a running tap is well known, or local warmth may be applied to the lower abdomen. However, in many instances the personality of the radiographer and the relationship of confidence and kindness which has been created are without doubt operative factors in swinging the balance from failure to success. Whatever the age of the patient, patience, encouragement and thought for their comfort are necessary.

The catheterized patient

Catheters are hollow tubes designed to be passed into cavities and passages of the body. The present section refers to the catheterization of the urinary bladder.

This may be undertaken for a variety of reasons – for example in cases of urinary retention when the patient cannot micturate naturally, a catheter is passed to relieve distension of the bladder. Catheterization is also done to allow the introduction of a contrast agent (as described in the previous section) to obtain an uncontaminated specimen of urine so that it may be bacteriologically examined, and to empty the bladder prior to special procedures such as cystoscopy or surgery to the pelvic organs. After pelvic surgery, a self-retaining catheter may be inserted in order to keep the bladder wall collapsed, or to prevent contamination of an operation area. This catheter may be connected to tubing which drains urine into a bottle or a plastic bag.

Catheterization of a patient will usually be done by a doctor or nurse although, again, some radiographers are now undertaking this after special training. It is very important for the student to realize that the bladder, unlike the rectum, is a sterile body cavity, and that infection of the urinary tract can occur extremely easily when instruments and catheters are passed into it.

Catheterization is therefore always undertaken most carefully with regard to the sterilization of the catheters, and their subsequent manipulation into the tract, so that no contamination occurs. Infection can occur from the catheter, the operator's hands, and the patient's skin. Some patients may require frequent catheterization (for example, paraplegic patients), and it is often the practice to give such patients chemotherapy in the form of drugs to combat any urinary infection which might arise.

It can be seen that preparing a trolley for catheterization of a patient involves the preparation of some sterile equipment. The technique of preparing a sterile trolley has already been described in an earlier section of this chapter, and need not be given again in detail. The methods for preserving sterility of the equipment which were stated in preparing for an intravenous injection should be meticulously applied to *any* procedure requiring sterile technique. They are therefore applicable in preparing a trolley for catheterization of the urinary bladder.

Various types of catheter are in use and any particular type of catheter will be available in different sizes. In modern practice catheters are usually made of plastic and are pre-sterilized by the manufacturer, each catheter in its own paper pack. Some may be of the self-retaining type.

It should be recognized that if the patient comes to the X-ray department with a catheter in place, then all parts of the catheter which are in the urethra and bladder or allow entry to the bladder (that is, all the *inside* of the catheter and some parts of the outside as well) are a sterile system. If the catheter is connected by rubber tubing to a container for drainage, then the inside of the tubing and of any container are included in the sterile system.

In handling and moving a catheterized patient, the radiographer must be careful at all times to see that the sterile system does not become open. If the catheter is closed with a spigot and the patient asks for the catheter to be released, then the spigot must be set down with care in a sterile container so that only its outer terminal is contaminated by the hands, or else it must be replaced with a fresh sterile one. The urine drained out of the catheter must be kept in a suitable container until the nurse in charge of the patient's ward can be notified of the amount and character of the urine passed.

If the catheter is connected to a tube and drainage container and it becomes disconnected while the patient is in the X-ray department, the catheter should be clamped, and the tubing and container returned intact to the ward with the patient, a report being given of what has occurred. If the catheter should come partly out, it should not be pushed back as this would mean insertion into the sterile area of a part of the catheter made unsterile by its extrusion. For the same reason no attempt should be made to replace a catheter which has come out completely; the ward should be notified of either of these occurrences. (Lowthian, 1989)

References

Chapman, S. & Nakielny, R. (1993) *A Guide to Radiological Procedures*, (pages 400–401), 3rd Edn., Baillière Tindall, London.

Lowthian, P. (1989) Catheters – preventing trauma. *Nursing Times*, May 24th, 85 (21), 73–5.

Maclennan, A. (1992) Analysing the care of the intravenous urogram patient. *Radiography Today*, 58 (656), 19–21.

Chapter 8
The Biliary Tract

A correctly exposed radiograph of the abdomen will reveal the outline of the liver, but the extra-hepatic parts of the biliary system are not normally demonstrated without the introduction of a contrast agent. On such a radiograph a common abnormality may be the appearance of gallstones, and it is to exclude or confirm the presence of these that the biliary tract is most frequently submitted to X-ray examination. Again, however, in many departments ultrasound is now the examination of first choice for the investigation of the biliary tract. The numbers of radiographic examinations of this region are thus falling.

Radiographic detection of gallstones

The radiopacity of gallstones, in a manner comparable with calculi in other anatomical systems, is related to the substances which compose them. Some gallstones contain a high proportion of calcium and these are readily detected on a plain radiograph. The student will soon appreciate, however, that they can vary in appearance. In some cases, even to an inexperienced eye they are easily recognizable as 'stones': they are large and circular or probably faceted in outline. Frequently their centres are radioparent in relation to the outer border and the impression of a hollow core or cavity is obtained. These stones may be so numerous as to fill more or less completely the entire gall bladder sac, and in this case the classic anatomical description of a 'pear shaped organ' comes to life on the radiograph. It is indeed apparent that we are looking at the gall bladder and that it contains a number of calculi. We need go no further for the diagnosis.

However, not all gallstones can be so readily identified from a plain film. If opaque, they may appear only as flecks or isolated spots of calcium in the right hypochondrium; they may overlie the renal outline, or be situated close to the lower ribs. In this case determination must be made that the opacities are in fact related to the gall bladder, and are not either renal calculi or calcified areas in costal cartilage.

Again, many gallstones do not contain calcium and are formed of cholesterol only. This substance is penetrated by X-rays and such stones

111

will not be apparent on a plain radiograph. In this circumstance too, a further procedure is necessary to exclude or confirm their presence: this procedure is the introduction of a contrast agent into the biliary tract.

Oral cholecystography

Oral cholecystography is a contrast examination of the gall bladder.

The student will have deduced from the term *oral* cholecystography that the contrast medium is taken by the mouth. It is therefore a simple procedure readily performed in outpatients. However, it requires a stringent preparation if it is to be fully successful and a considerable amount of time to complete all its stages. The examination has three sections.

(1) A preliminary radiograph is taken before administration of the contrast agent; we may label this control film (or films) as occurring on Day 1.
(2) Radiographs – sometimes described as *repletion* radiographs – are taken after administration of the contrast agent, most usually about 12–16 hours later; we may label this phase of the examination as occurring on Day 2.
(3) A minimum of one radiograph is exposed some 8 to 30 minutes after the patient has taken a meal containing fat. This part of the procedure follows immediately on (2) above and thus also occurs on Day 2.

Preparation of the patient

Each stage of the examination requires the patient to submit to certain preliminaries.

The preliminary radiograph

When making the appointment for the preliminary radiograph the patient should be told something of the full examination, particularly the facts that it will necessitate his visiting the department on two consecutive days and that the demand on his time will be markedly greater on the second day than on the first. In some instances a visit on a third morning may be necessary. The preparation for the preliminary radiograph is usually the department's routine for abdominal X-ray examination which – with some of its difficulties – has been discussed in Chapter 5.

For cholecystography good preparation is particularly desirable. Its absence frequently increases to a great degree the time required to complete the examination satisfactorily. The reason for this is that intestinal gas shadows can simulate transradiant (cholesterol) stones if they happen to overlie the image of the opacified gall bladder. On the radiograph taken following ingestion of the contrast medium both entities appear as rounded dark areas. To make the differential diagnosis it is necessary to obtain at least one radiograph in which the gall bladder is seen to lie clear of any intestinal shadows.

Evidently this may involve considerable extension of the examination while various radiographic projections are applied, with consequent loss of time for the patient and increased demand upon the department. If it can be avoided by adequate measures in the first place, it is in everyone's interest – our own not least – to make the initial preparation of the patient as efficient as possible.

It is recognized, however, that it is not always possible to obtain the ideal. In the case of in-patients it is not difficult to repeat the process of preparation, should the first radiograph reveal accumulations of abdominal gas. Where outpatients are concerned it is less easy to arrange further preparation and renewed attendance in the department, and because of this it is usual to accept the first result, unless conditions are seen to be really extremely unsatisfactory.

Day 2 – Post-contrast radiographs

Once a satisfactory preliminary radiograph has been obtained, the patient receives instruction on how to use the contrast agent. Generally, the patient will be asked to take this during the evening of Day 1 and consequently they will require to know what they may – or may not – eat during the intervening hours.

There is usually little difficulty about lunch. This should be a light meal and – whenever appropriate – should maintain the patient on the low-residue diet which they may have followed on the previous day. However, a routine commonly followed does allow the patient to take some fat.

Any evening meal taken at this stage of oral cholecystography must occur before ingestion of the contrast agent. There are three possibilities regarding it:

(1) The meal should *contain fat*. This will contract the gall bladder and empty it of bile in readiness for the reception of the contrast agent.
(2) The meal should be *free of fat*. This will allow the contrast agent to mix readily with the normal bile content of the system.
(3) The meal – which should be light and preferably leave little intestinal residue – may be otherwise of almost any character, to a patient's taste. This unusual freedom reflects a general inconclusiveness of evidence that either abstention from, or adherence to, an intake of fat materially affects successful visualization of the gall bladder during oral cholecystography.

Student radiographers in consequence are likely to encounter any of several variations on the suggested lines; or may find that different methods are tried from time to time within their own departments. Whatever is the accepted practice, or eventual decision, the radiographer's responsibility is to give a patient specific instruction about the meal which they are allowed to take.

If the meal in question is to include fat, then the patient may be told to have something fried on the menu. Unfortunately sufferers from diseases of the gall bladder are often intolerant of fat and will protest that they never eat fried food as it brings on their pain. In the circumstances an insistence that they do so will be received with understandable reluctance and opposition. More acceptable may be a request that the evening meal should include an egg, bread and butter and a milky drink.

Patients usually are familiar with some foods which contain fat and have no difficulty in recognizing a suitable item for the menu when instructed that fat should be taken. It is the second (fat-free) category of meal which is the more likely to cause confusion. It is not enough to give the patient merely the negative instruction, 'You must not eat anything containing fat'. They may not be sufficiently educated in dietetics to recognize that milk contains fat, and will almost certainly rely on the favoured cup of tea or coffee to sustain them.

It is much better to amplify the instruction to avoid fat with positive details of what food is allowed. The following suggestions may be made.

- Any lean meat,
- White fish (steamed),
- Smoked haddock,
- Fresh or grilled tomatoes,
- Garden peas, though these, perhaps, are better avoided as they tend to produce gas during digestion,
- Boiled potatoes,
- Fruit of any kind, stewed or fresh according to taste,
- Fruit drinks,
- Tea or coffee must be taken black or with *skimmed* milk only: they are probably better avoided.

Taking the contrast medium

Various agents for oral cholecystography are available and in general use (see point (2) under Iodine Preparations, Chapter 3). A tablet and a capsule are the two most common presentations, of which the patient is required to take a number varying from six to twelve at one time. One product is available also as a powder which is taken as a suspension in fluid. Apart from any clinical feature, this may offer certain advantages to a patient who – as many people are – is a poor swallower of tablets. In any department the choice of medium to be generally used is a matter of radiological opinion, based on experience of clinical results.

A comparable diversity exists for methods of dose distribution, on which no uniform clinical agreement even now has been reached. The following techniques are well established in practice, the first being the one most frequently employed.

(1) A single dose (3 g) of the selected contrast agent (e.g. 'Telepaque') is taken on the evening of Day 1. In the case of a heavy patient the dose may be increased to 4.5 g.
(2) Two doses on consecutive days; for example, the evening of Day 1 and the early morning of Day 2.
(3) A fractionated dose over several hours (Days 1 and 2).

The most usual timing of the radiograph on Day 2 is to bring the patient to the X-ray department between nine and ten in the morning, some 12 to 15 hours following ingestion of the contrast agent: this is, he will have taken a light evening meal of the appropriate kind at possibly 6 or 7 PM, followed by the specified medium at 8.0 to 9.0 PM. Tablets of capsules should be swallowed whole and one at a time with a draught of water. If the contrast medium is in powder form, its container should be filled with water and shaken until a suspension is formed. This should then be swallowed in one or two gulps, followed by a glass of fruit squash or water.

After this the patient must fast until the X-ray examination on the following morning. If he is thirsty, he may have a fruit drink or water according to his taste. In some instances, particularly when frying is the method of cooking, merely the smell of food has been thought to cause contraction and emptying of the gall bladder, with consequent failure of the examination. However, though taste and smell have a stimulating effect on the gall bladder, in themselves they do not lead to evacuation of bile. Some radiologists prefer the patient to abstain from smoking during this period.

Where it is departmental practice to take the radiographs a little later in the day, or where a special arrangement is made to suit some individual convenience, appropriate adjustments to the whole scheme of events of course will be needed. However, it should be kept in mind when making any particular alterations that it is hardly a suitable arrangement which would require the patient to take the contrast medium in the middle of the night. Consequently any appointments for the afternoon should be carefully considered.

Care of the patient

It is the responsibility of the radiographer to discover from the patient whether any untoward effects have resulted from taking the contrast agent.

In the medium used for cholecystography the opacity is due to iodine. The student should be already familiar with the radiopaque nature of this element and will know how often it is employed to obtain radiographic contrast in a large number of procedures. In the previous chapter reference has been made to the sensitivity of certain individuals to this substance, and occasionally in the course of cholecystography the allergic type of reaction is encountered. However, it is rather unusual and when it does occur is seldom worse than an uncomfortable urticaria and perhaps a general malaise of a few hours' duration.

Much more common are gastrointestinal disturbances which essentially are reactions, not to the iodine content of the preparation, but to the complex salt which 'carries' the iodine molecule. The patient may experience nausea and vomiting, or diarrhoea, sometimes to a prostrating degree. In this regard, however, the modern contrast agents for cholecystography are generally much better tolerated than were their forerunners.

These reactions, when they occur, may prevent concentration of the agent in the gall bladder and lead to the impression that dysfunction is present. It is therefore important to ask the patient specifically about any ill results. It is surprising how many patients believe that the purpose of the contrast agent was to induce bowel action and that their diarrhoea was intended to occur. In those cases when the patient has suffered from diarrhoea after taking the medium and no filling of the gall bladder is detected on the repletion series of radiographs, it is usual to repeat the examination on the following day, possibly with the use of another oral cholecystographic agent. The patient should remain on a fat-free menu until after completion of this further examination.

The object of the post-contrast radiographs is twofold:

(1) To obtain a firm diagnosis of the presence of gallstones;
(2) To assess function of the gall bladder – that is, its ability to concentrate and store bile.

On these radiographs opaque calculi will remain in constant relation to the opacified gall bladder. Cholesterol stones, which cannot be detected on the plain film owing to their radioparency, will now appear as dark areas (negative shadows) superimposed on the image of the gall bladder: sometimes, if they are numerous and small, they adopt a characteristic string formation when a radiograph is taken in the erect posture. Reference has already been made to the possibility of confusing intestinal gas with these cholesterol stones and to the significance of good preparation of the patient in this connection.

The fatty meal
When the second part of the examination has been satisfactorily performed,

the final stage completes the assessment of gall bladder function. It may obtain visualization of the common bile duct if this has not been apparent on the earlier series, and will show calculi maintaining their relation to the now contracted and diminished gall bladder shadow.

As a preliminary to this last stage of cholecystography, the patient must take a meal containing fat. In most cases, for convenience sake this 'meal' is actually a synthetic product containing fat in a concentrated form given as a drink.

One of these is a fluid of milky appearance and is not unattractive to the eye as when poured from the container it develops a slight frothy 'head'. Another has the appearance of *café au lait* and a taste suggestive of coffee. The average subject should not find either nauseous to take in a small quantity. It must be borne in mind, however, that many patients undergoing cholecystography are readily sickened by fat and there is a definite psychological advantage in presenting this draught as attractively as possible.

When the patient is given a meal in the department he should be provided with peaceful and relatively private surroundings in which to take it.

Alternatively to the use of synthetic products, the diet kitchen may be asked to supply an appropriate light meal. In this case the choice of food can be important. A glass of milk and some buttered toast are likely to prove more appetizing then fried fare of any kind.

Intravenous cholangiography

In this radiological investigation a contrast medium is introduced intravenously to the biliary tract. Its subsequent appearance in the biliary system is not dependent – as oral cholecystography generally is – upon a functioning gall bladder, but upon excretory function of the liver. It is therefore suitable for examination of the hepatic ducts in subjects in whom the gall bladder has been removed; or for visualization of the gall bladder itself, when oral cholecystography has failed to produce or has shown inadequate radiological evidence of function. It is recommended that an interval of 4 to 7 days should elapse between oral and intravenous cholecystography. This examination is rapidly being superseded by ultrasound in the majority of centres.

Preparation of the patient

Considerations which apply to the preparation of patients for intravenous cholangiography are closely similar to those already discussed in relation to oral cholecystography. This examination can be completed during one visit to the department, since following the intravenous injection the biliary passages are usually well visualized within 30 minutes, and filling of the gall bladder is obtained in a period varying from 45 minutes to 3 hours. The patient should be given some indication that he is likely to be retained in the department throughout the morning or afternoon.

Apart from the general principles discussed in Chapter 5, some diversity of opinion exists as to the best preparation for intravenous cholangiography. A typical preparation might be:

(1) A light low-fat diet on the day before the examination;
(2) A fat-free breakfast on the morning of the examination.

Intravenous cholangiography has been successfully undertaken without any specialized preparation of the patient at all in many instances. During the course of the examination itself, nothing either to eat or drink should be given, nor should the patient smoke after the injection has been made.

In some cases preparation of the patient may include the use of certain drugs to modify the activity of the sphincter of Oddi. For example, 20 to 50 mg pethidine given intravenously will cause immediate contraction of the sphincter and thus retention of bile within the biliary system. This should result in improved radiopacity of the gall bladder on the introduction of the contrast agent.

Preparation of the trolley

Introduction of the contrast agent is effected through an intravenous drip infusion. The trolley to be prepared requires the following items.

Sterile

- An intravenous drip infusion set (see Fig. 8.1),
- 'Sterets' for skin cleansing,
- 'Butterfly' needles or cannulae.

Non-sterile

- Contrast agent (e.g. 'Biliscopin'),
- Water in a dressings bowl to warm the contrast agent,
- A bowl containing cotton wool swabs,
- A few small 'plaster' dressings for the skin wound,
- A roll of narrow adhesive tape,
- A pair of scissors,
- A tourniquet,
- A small sandbag or padded board for support of the arm,
- A receiver in case of vomiting.

A dripstand also is necessary and should be on hand before the procedure is begun.

Care of the patient

The intravenous drip infusion will be set up by either a radiologist or some other medically qualified person (see Direct Cholangiography, below).

At this stage of the procedure, the patient should have received a brief and reassuring explanation of what the examination involves. Reassurance should be given as to its ease and simplicity. In the previous chapter reference was made to reactions which may appear following the administration of radiological contrast agents containing iodine. The possibility of these exists, whatever may be the procedure concerned and – should ill effects occur – naturally they will prove more severe if the iodine content of the medium is high and the dose large.

The treatment of adverse reactions is discussed fully in Chapter 7. The most likely occurrences of course are minor and transient: flushing of the skin; sneezing and coughing; nausea and vomiting. For these effects, a comforting presence, warm covering and adequate ventilation are all that should be needed.

The patient having intravenous infusion of fluid

In various cases as part of the patient's treatment it may be necessary to give him fluid by a method other than oral administration. This may be because the patient is unable to take anything by mouth owing to such causes as a mouth injury, surgery to the gastrointestinal tract, or a comatose state. It may be that the patient *can* take fluid by mouth, but it is required that a severe fluid loss (due to vomiting or diarrhoea or some other cause) should be quickly replaced in order to restore the correct fluid balance of the body. If the patient requires additional blood in order to make up loss by haemorrhage, transfusion of blood is similarly undertaken by an intravenous route.

A patient receiving such an infusion has an intravenous needle fixed into a vein usually in the arm. This needle is connected to a container which is hung upside down from a hooked stand above the patient. Not far below the container, the tubing which connects it to the needle is interrupted by insertion of a drop counter, in which the fluid can be seen dripping down the needle. Above the drop counter, between it and the container, is a tubing clip which regulates the rate of flow.

In modern practice the equipment for giving a drip infusion is made up into a basic pack and is disposable. This disposable equipment comes with its inner parts pre-sterilized by the manufacturer – that is, there is a sterile pathway for the flow of fluid through it. Some parts of the exterior of the equipment are sterile and are protected by sheaths which are removed before use.

The first part of the equipment (Fig. 8.1) consists of two transparent plastic chambers set one above the other. The upper is the filter chamber and it has in it, suspended from its top edge, a filtering sac through which the fluid which is to be infused must pass as it enters the chamber; the lower one is the drip chamber and contains a float ball. This float ball closes the exit from the chamber in the event of its having been allowed to become empty.

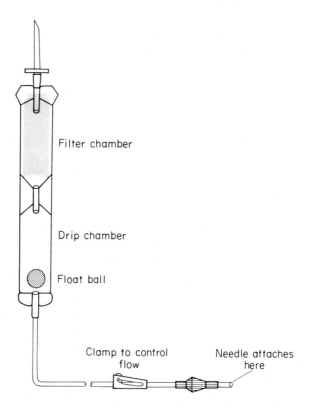

Fig. 8.1 Disposable equipment for giving an intravenous (drip) infusion.

The upper chamber has projecting above it a piercing needle enclosed by a sheath. In use, the sheath is removed from the needle and the piercing needle is then pushed into the infusion bag which contains the prescribed fluid to be given to the patient.

When the bag is suspended on the dripstand, the fluid fills the filter chamber by gravity and drips through a narrow tube communicating with the drip chamber: 15 drops will be approximately equivalent to 1 ml of fluid.

A length (about 1.5 metres) of plastic tubing leads from the bottom of the drip chamber. The lower end of this tubing is protected by a sheath which is removed so that the tubing can be attached to an intravenous needle for insertion into the vein that is to be used for the infusion. The plastic tubing carries a device which can be used to control the flow of fluid along it. In Fig. 8.1 the sheaths protecting the piercing needle and the lower end of the plastic tube have been removed.

The second part of the equipment (not shown in Fig. 8.1) is an air-inlet assembly to allow air into the suspended container so that the fluid running out is replaced by air. The air-inlet assembly is a short (about 40 cm) length of narrow plastic tubing with a short-bevelled needle at one end and a small wire hook attached to the other end, which is open; both ends are protected by sheaths which are removed before use. The needle on the air-inlet tube enters the fluid-container and when the container is suspended the air-inlet tube is hooked up in a suitable position by means of the little hook attached to it. Air can then enter the container through the plastic tubing.

The radiographer has no responsibility for altering or setting the rate of flow of an intravenous infusion, but while dealing with such a patient should observe certain points. It must be seen that the needle does not become dislodged from its site in the vein, and that in moving the patient the tubing is not kinked or compressed so that the rate of flow is obstructed.

The patient's arm may be bandaged to a splint so that they may move it without disturbance of the needle, but some care will nevertheless be necessary to see that the needle is not pulled or jerked out of place. While with the patient, the radiographer should observe the drop counter or drip chamber every so often to see that the fluid is continuing to flow properly.

There are several possible causes for an infusion to cease to flow. Some of them (and the remedial actions to be taken) are set out in Table 8.1.

The radiographer should look at the patient's arm. If the needle has dislodged itself from the vein and is still in the tissues, there will be a flow of fluid into the tissues of the arm and a swelling will develop around the needle site.

If the needle comes right out of the patient's arm, the tubing clip must be used to clamp off the flow of fluid, and pressure should be exerted for a few minutes at the injection site to prevent extravasation of blood into the tissues. All these occurrences – cessation of the flow of fluid, suspicion that the needle has been moved out of the vein, or total dislodgement of the needle from the arm – must be reported immediately to the ward staff.

In moving the X-ray equipment, the radiographer must notice the position of the suspended container and take care not to strike it with the X-ray tube head. The wheeled stand can be moved about a little if care is taken to see that no strain is put on the tubing, but the container should not be

Table 8.1 Problems which may occur with an intravenous (drip) infusion.

Infusion stops because	Remedied by
1 Tubing is kinked	Straightening the tubing
2 There is restriction above the site of injection	Making sure that bandages and clothing on the limb are not tight
3 The head of pressure is too low	Raising the bottle
4 The needle may: *a* be against the wall of the vein	*a* straightening limb and adjusting needle, but *not* advancing or withdrawing it
b have punctured the wall of the vein	*b* medical officer who will start infusion in another vein
c be blocked by a clot	*c* aspiration by a medical officer using a sterile syringe
5 The vein is in spasm	Stroking a finger along the vein above the injection site
6 The vein is thrombosed	medical officer who will start infusion again

lowered from its position above the patient. If it is seen to be nearly empty the attention of the ward staff should be drawn to this fact.

The method of intravenous drip infusion may be used to give a radiographic contrast agent, as described above.

Direct cholangiography

Those examinations of the biliary tract which have been described (oral cholecystography and intravenous cholangiography) depend on certain physiological functions for the introduction of the radiological contrast agent to the site of the examination. In distinction from these procedures the biliary tree may be directly injected with a suitable contrast agent, once surgery has made the ducts accessible. The purpose of such direct investigation is to ensure that – with the gall bladder itself – the surgeon has removed all biliary calculi and that none remains in the extra-hepatic or intraheptic parts of the system; thus a demonstration of the entire biliary tree is the criterion of radiographic success.

Injection of the ducts may be made immediately at operation (operative cholangiography); or a few days later through the tube left for drainage purposes in the wound during a short period following cholecystectomy (T-tube cholangiography). Mechanically we need hardly differentiate the procedures; both entail a direct filling of the same anatomical pathways. A

water-soluble contrast agent such as 'Conray 280' is used and in neither case
is a special preparation of the patient required. Both of these procedures are
again reducing in numbers as laparoscopic (*keyhole*) surgery becomes more
widespread.

Students may meet some differences in the process of administration of
the contrast agents. Two methods of operative cholangiography, for
instance, have been described.

(1) The common bile duct is punctured with a curved 20 gauge spinal
    needle and 20 ml of the contrast agent are injected as a single bolus.
    Three radiographs are then taken at 2 minute intervals.
(2) The cystic duct is cannulated with a catheter and radiographs are
    taken at 2 minute intervals, after injection of 3 ml, 6 ml, and 11 ml of
    contrast agent. Sometimes 1 mg glucagon is given intravenously 3
    minutes before the first injection, in order to decrease resistance to bile
    flow.

Percutaneous transhepatic cholangiography

Transhepatic cholangiography is another technique for introducing contrast
into the biliary passages by direct injection and is again to be distinguished
from the physiological oral or intravenous methods earlier considered.

In this difficult procedure the biliary system is entered through one of the
dilated ducts in the liver itself which is penetrated by a needle inserted
through the abdominal wall; often although not invariably at a site 1–2 cm
below and to the right of the xiphisternum.

Many radiologists prefer to use a needle-catheter, which is potentially a
safer instrument. This is a short length of polythene tubing about 1.5 mm in
diameter which is tailored to suit the needle, one end being tapered to a close
fit. The other extremity is flanged and carries a collar and adaptor with a tap,
similar to the arrangements required by the Seldinger technique for
aortography. The length of the catheter is a little less than that of the needle,
which is of the order of 12–15 cm.

The needle is first passed down the catheter and the composite tool used
to enter the liver. As soon as this has occurred the needle is at once withdrawn, leaving the catheter alone in place. The operator then pulls gently on
the catheter at the same time as he applies suction at its free end by means of
an attached syringe, until he sees by entry of bile into the syringe that the
catheter tip is lying within a bile duct. After this the injection of contrast
agent (for example 20–50 ml of 'Conray 280') is made under fluoroscopic
control and films are taken as needed. In some cases it may be possible to
guide a catheter past the site of the biliary obstruction.

Percutaneous transhepatic cholangiography is undertaken when other methods of investigating the biliary system either have failed or have had a doubtful result. These patients most probably have a long-standing jaundice, due to either duct obstruction or damage of the liver cells, and thus have experienced a disabling illness for a considerable time.

Preparation on the ward of such a patient is likely to contain the following provisions.

(1) The patient should have signed a consent form before being brought to the X-ray department.
(2) Any treatment with an anti-coagulant will be stopped.
(3) Blood clotting factors will be checked and corrected, if necessary.
(4) Vitamin K will be given on the day before the examination (and again on the day after the examination).

The second, third and fourth of these measures are considered necessary because jaundice is a condition which abnormally lowers the level of prothrombin in the blood plasma: blood clotting power is thus deficient. The administration of vitamin K helps to maintain the prothrombin level.

Following the X-ray examination, immediate care of the patient entails half-hourly checks on pulse and blood pressure during a period of four hours. In the longer term, treatment with a broad spectrum antibiotic may be instituted, since there is a risk of septicaemia; but this prophylaxis is not in the hands of the X-ray department, of course, and not the concern of this book.

Endoscopic retrograde cholangiopancreatography

Endoscopic retrograde cholangiopancreatography is the descriptive name of a diagnostic procedure which radiographers generally recognize under the more convenient – though less explicit – title of ERCP. In common with other investigations this one is directed at the excretory apparatus of the liver; but as well it permits visualization of the pancreatic duct and is often the better diagnostician of a pancreatic lesion than is medical ultrasound.

During ERCP, an endoscope is passed via the mouth, oesophagus and stomach into the duodenum. The sphincter of Oddi – the circular muscle surrounding the lower part of the bile duct which includes the ampulla and the terminus of the pancreatic duct – is cannulated. A radiological contrast agent is then introduced and the ducts are studied fluoroscopically; records and analyses of these images may be made by any of the usual means but the emphasis of the procedure is more on endoscopy accompanied by fluoroscopy than on a formal series of radiographs.

Care of the patient and preparation of the trolley

Typically, preparation of both the patient – who must be starved for 6 hours beforehand – and a trolley lay-out for ERCP is a responsibility of nursing staff on a gastroenterological ward or unit. When brought to the X-ray department, the patient should have had the procedure explained and should have signed the usual consent form.

Clearly, the trolley will include an endoscope and its accessories, as well as the means to premedicate the patient (diazepam is a suitable sedative) and to give the radiological contrast agent (Conray 280 would be an appropriate choice). The use of a sedative will allow the patient to co-operate in the introduction of the endoscope, tolerate the examination well – and remember very little afterwards. It is usual for the enterologist to be assisted during passage of the endoscope and the introduction of the radiological contrast agent. The patient should be in position on the fluoroscopic/ radiographic table throughout, since the enterologist may wish from time to time to check the location of the endoscope externally by means of a fluoroscopic inspection. It is the responsibility of the radiographer present to ensure that the radiological equipment is functioning correctly and to operate it at the doctor's request.

After the examination the patient must not be allowed to eat or drink until sensation has returned to the pharyngeal area, as otherwise the patient is in danger of choking. Observations may be undertaken for up to 6 hours afterwards.

Further reading

Chapman, S. & Nakielny, R. (1993) *A Guide to Radiological Procedures*, 3rd Edn., Baillière Tindall, London.

Chapter 9
The Respiratory Tract

Bronchography

Bronchography is the procedure during which a radiological contrast agent is introduced to the respiratory system immediately before exposure of an appropriate series of radiographs. It is in less frequent use than formerly, partly because of a decline in the incidence of bronchiectasis; to the diagnosis and treatment of which bronchography was often applied and largely because other imaging methods, in particular computed tomography, can now give the same diagnostic information in a rather less invasive and unpleasant fashion.

In the case of a patient undergoing bronchoscopy, and if bronchography is part of the diagnostic plan, a catheter can be positioned easily by means of the bronchoscope, and the reader is referred to Chapter 8 and the section on endoscopic retrograde cholangiopancreatography for comparable patient care details.

Care of patients with respiratory difficulties

Whilst we may no longer undertake many contrast agent examinations of the respiratory tract, it is the case that radiographers have to deal with many patients with conditions of the respiratory tract which require special care and attention. Let us consider these conditions now.

Oxygen therapy

All the living cells of the body demand oxygen, and normally enough can be supplied by the act of respiration in ordinary atmospheric air. In certain circumstances, however, there will be reduced oxygen in the blood – a condition known as anoxaemia. It may show itself in the patient's face by blueness of the nose and the tips of the ears and about the mouth, and the blue coloration will also be detected in the patient's nails. This blue tinge is known as cyanosis.

Administration of oxygen

Oxygen is given to patients in the treatment of conditions in which normal supply of oxygen to the tissue-cells is not being maintained. In normal physiology, oxygen is carried to the cells by the haemoglobin in the circulating blood. Failure to maintain the normal supply can be caused by:

(1) Lack of haemoglobin so that there is no haemoglobin to take up the oxygen;
(2) Interference with the processes by which haemoglobin takes up oxygen so that although haemoglobin and oxygen may both be present the oxygen is not taken up;
(3) Failure of the blood in circulation so that there is no haemoglobin circulating to carry the oxygen to the body's tissues.

Oxygen may be given to a patient to treat the following conditions.

- Severe anaemia (not enough haemoglobin).
- Shock (blood is not circulating well).
- Severe loss of blood (not enough haemoglobin).
- Circulatory failure (blood not circulating).
- Respiratory failure. ⎫ In all these three conditions the oxygenating
- Pulmonary oedema. ⎬ process that should take place within the lungs
- Pneumonia. ⎭ is impaired.
- Carbon monoxide poisoning (loss of haemoglobin through chemical combination).

Patients who require oxygen are in two categories of need as follows.

(1) Those who need an amount which is strictly controlled. Such patients are most often chronic bronchitics with respiratory failure. For these patients the concentration of oxygen must not exceed 24–26%, the aim being to raise the blood content of oxygen to an acceptable level which is below the point at which the respiratory centre in the brain is depressed: if this centre is unstimulated the patient's breathing becomes very shallow and he may pass into a coma.
(2) Those who need simply a high percentage of oxygen (30–60%) which is intended to raise the blood content of oxygen high enough to relieve symptoms. These patients have a low level of arterial oxygen which is not due to respiratory failure. It has been suggested, however, that long periods of administration of high percentages of oxygen (50% or more) should be avoided as they may be toxic (Higgins, 1990).

So there are many conditions in which the patient can benefit by the administration of oxygen and there are various ways in which he can be enabled to breathe an additional amount in the air which he inhales.

The oxygen supply

Oxygen is supplied commercially compressed in cylinders. Cylinders of medical gases are standardized as to size and colour, being provided in a certain range of sizes and in a colour individual to the gas contained in the cylinder. Oxygen cylinders are *black with white shoulders and upper part* where the outlet valve is situated. The name or the symbol O_2 (and sometimes both) may be seen painted upon the outside of the cylinder. It is obviously important at all times to be able to distinguish a cylinder readily and quickly, so that the risk of the patient being given the wrong gas in a moment of crisis is reduced (see Fig. 9.1).

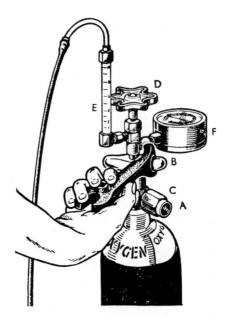

Fig. 9.1 An oxygen cylinder fitted with a fine adjustment valve. The illustration shows: A, main tap for turning on flow of oxygen; B, wing nut for attaching regulator, etc., to the cylinder (this nut may be loosened with a special spanner); C, lock nut; D, fine adjustment valve; E, flowmeter; F, pressure gauge. *(Reproduced by courtesy of Baillière, Tindall & Cox Ltd.)*

In hospitals oxygen is piped directly to the wards and certain departments from a central supply in the basement. Oxygen is then available at the patient's bedside by means of this pipeline. It is, however, less likely that the X-ray department will be included entirely in this arrangement where it exists for the wards; sometimes one or two rooms in a department may be equipped with piped gases which would include oxygen. The department must therefore maintain as part of its emergency equipment complete apparatus for delivering oxygen to the patient.

The oxygen cylinder and regulating valve

For use, the oxygen cylinder has attached to it a regulating valve. This fitment has a threaded end which goes into the upper end of the oxygen cylinder, and is locked in place by means of a nut which may be of the wing type. This nut is tightened by a special spanner which is also used to turn the main tap on the cylinder which releases the oxygen flow.

The regulating valve incorporates a pressure gauge which shows the amount of oxygen present in the cylinder, and a regulator which can be adjusted to control the flow of oxygen. A flowmeter which shows the amount of oxygen being used is another feature of the cylinder fitting, and such a meter may be either a dial or a dry bobbin type; in the latter case a bobbin moves up and down inside a glass tube which is calibrated with scale markings, the height of the bobbin against the markings indicating the flow. Both the dial and the bobbin type of flowmeter record the flow in litres per minute.

The regulating valve fitment, with its pressure gauge and flowmeter, is attached to the oxygen cylinder (as has been explained) by means of the threaded end which inserts into the valve opening at the head of the cylinder. Before this is done, the main tap of the cylinder should be opened a little and some of the oxygen allowed to escape. This will dislodge any small impediments which may have collected around the valve opening. With the valve closed again, the threaded end of the regulator fitting is inserted and tightened in place by means of the nut for the purpose. (At this stage the regulator controlling the flow of oxygen through the flowmeter should be in the 'off' position.) The main tap on the side of the regulator is then turned on. The pressure gauge recording the contents of the cylinder will register 'Full' when the cylinder is a new one.

The cylinder is now ready to supply oxygen to the patient when the regulator valve is opened to produce the required rate of flow as registered on the flowmeter.

The cylinder with its regulator fitment and meters constitute the apparatus necessary to *deliver* oxygen. In order to administer it to the patient certain further equipment is needed. The nature of this will depend on the method of administration.

Methods of administering oxygen

There are various ways of administering oxygen to patients, as set out in Table 9.1 and as further considered below.

Any of the four ways described in the table may be used for continuous oxygen therapy when the patient is in the ward or in intensive care. The choice of mask depends on whether the patient needs oxygen in a strictly controlled quantity or in a high concentration. If the oxygen is to be strictly

Table 9.1 Methods of administering oxygen.

Methods	Devices used	Notes
1 Masks of various types	(a) Polymask Disposable. Essentially a double plastic bag with oxygen passing between the layers and holes in the plastic so that patient breathes air mixed with oxygen. Delivers 30–50% at 4 litres per minute. (b) Edinburgh Disposable mask. Air enters as well as oxygen. Delivers low concentrations, 35% at 3 litres per minute (c) Ventimask Disposable mask with a rigid base. Air enters as well as oxygen. Delivers 25% at 4 litres per minute or higher concentrations at other flow rates.	Masks are the only method to give close control of the amount given. Patient must remove the mask to talk, eat, drink.
2 Intranasal tubes	(a) Catheters which extend 2 cm into the nostrils, one in each nostril coming to a Y junction below the nose with a single attachment to the oxygen supply (b) Cannulae inserted 7–10 cm to reach the nasopharynx.	For these catheters the patient must be able to keep the mouth closed. The longer nasal cannulae are not comfortable. The necessity to keep the mouth closed is removed.
3 Tents	Plastic tent hung over the bed and extending down the sides which is filled with oxygen.	Tents are used for adults only when masks and nasal catheters cannot be tolerated. Tents may cause feelings of isolation, and patients need reassurance about this.
4 Incubators for neonatal babies	Incubators as used in intensive care baby units.	Tents and incubators are widely used for children

controlled it must be given by a mask: a tent or the intranasal method must not be used. Tents and incubators are used widely for babies and children. For an adult who cannot tolerate a mask or nasal catheters, a tent is a necessity. For emergency use in the X-ray department only a mask can be applied, the other methods being unsuitable to this application.

A high concentration of dry oxygen is very irritating to the respiratory tract and some method of humidifying the oxygen is often necessary.

Several sorts of equipment are available to do this. When a plastic mask is used, the patient's breath within the mask and incoming air will sufficiently moisten the oxygen and then no special apparatus is needed.

Oxygen masks

Modern oxygen masks are usually disposable and made of plastic which may be rigid or not according to type.

In the X-ray department the mask to be used is often non-rigid. It is a disposable mask of light transparent plastic on a wire frame. It fits over the patient's nose and mouth, and is held in place with narrow cords over the ears (see Fig. 9.2). The mask consists of a double plastic bag, oxygen passing from the cylinder (again by means of rubber or polythene connecting tubing) into the space between the inner and outer layers of the bag. The inner layer has two holes which allow the oxygen to enter the inside of the bag and reach the patient. Some moist expired air goes into the space between the layers and humidifies the incoming oxygen, so this type of mask also acts as a humidifier.

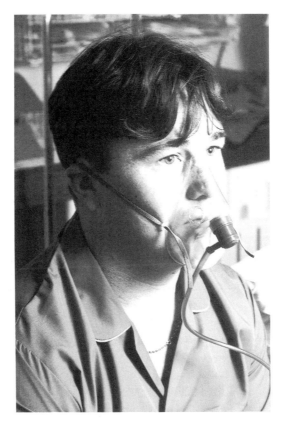

Fig. 9.2 Patient wearing an oxygen mask.

Oxygen administration by nasal catheter

In this method two fine rubber tubes are passed into the patient's nasal passages, one up each nostril. The two tubes from the nostrils are connected by a Y-shaped junction to a single tube which receives oxygen from the cylinder bubbled through a bottle of water.

The oxygen tent

There are several types of oxygen tent in use which may show variety in detail but are similar in basic construction. The tent is of light transparent plastic material fixed to a frame, the whole assembly being mounted on wheels so that it can be wheeled into position over the patient's bed. The canopy of the tent is capacious enough to allow its free edges to be tucked in at front, sides, and back, so that the patient is totally enclosed. Oxygen is fed into the upper part of the tent.

The tent has certain features of design to prevent the air inside becoming too hot and damp, cooling of the air usually being done by passing it through an ice box. Some tents incorporate forced circulation of the oxygen and improvement of ventilation by means of a motor.

Maintenance of emergency oxygen equipment

The oxygen cylinder (on a wheeled stand so that it can be readily transported), the regulator valve and meters fitted to it, and a mask for administering oxygen are important parts of emergency equipment in the X-ray department. They should be maintained assembled and ready for use. Large departments will certainly have more than one set of such equipment.

Each oxygen cylinder should be daily checked to see that it is full; if it is nearly empty it must be replaced by a full one, and not left until it is nearly exhausted. When the cylinder is being changed, the main escape valve should be turned off before the regulator fitting is removed.

The oxygen key or spanner which opens the main escape valve on the cylinder should be kept attached to it with a tape so that it is to hand for instant use. The mask should be inspected regularly to see that it is in good order, and without holes or defects which would allow escape of oxygen intended for the patient.

A general review of the responsibilities of a radiographer in regard to the administration of oxygen in the department includes the following. The radiographer must ensure that:

(1) The cylinder is the correct black-and-white labelled oxygen cylinder;
(2) The cylinder is available and can be brought to the patient without delay;

(3) The cylinder is clean, dust-free and regularly checked for function;
(4) The cylinder has an indicating label to show it as *full*, or *empty*, or *in use*;
(5) The cylinder has with it a key or valve spanner and that the valve is open;
(6) There is a second companion cylinder marked *full*;
(7) There are masks and appropriate tubing available for immediate use.

Observations to be made

If you are attending a patient who is receiving oxygen you must maintain certain observations of the patient and of the equipment.

For the patient, you must observe:

(1) Colour;
(2) Respiration;
(3) Pulse;
(4) Any distress signals such as restlessness, obvious anxiety, greater effort in respiration.

For the equipment you must observe:

(1) The flow rate;
(2) The tubing for broken connections, kinks, obstructions;
(3) Any disturbance to the mask, which must be correctly placed over nose and mouth.

Risks associated with oxygen therapy

There are certain risks and unfavourable aspects associated with the giving of oxygen to patients. These are listed below.

(1) Fire. This is an ever-present and most serious hazard. Oxygen while not itself inflammable is a strong supporter of combustion and any material which burns in air will burn very much more rapidly in an atmosphere of air with an increased oxygen content. The risk must always be remembered and the necessary precautions must be observed strictly. These are:
(a) No smoking;
(b) No naked lights;
(c) No electrical equipment (which includes X-ray equipment) operating when oxygen is in use;
(d) No oil, no grease, no spirit on the equipment or on the patient;
(e) No metal or wind-up mechanical toys for a child;
(f) Remember the possibility of static electric discharge and consider

clothing and bedding (nylon is risky) and hair (combing and brushing dry hair) as sources of electric charge through friction and so the sources of sparks.

(2) Irritation of the membranes of the bronchi and the alveoli of the lungs from high concentrations of dry oxygen.

(3) The dangers of giving 100% concentration of oxygen (that is, there is no mixture with air) with the possible results of:
   (a) Convulsions;
   (b) Ear-ache;
   (c) Pains in the nasal sinuses;
   (d) Damage to the lungs (Higgins, 1990).

(4) The risk to babies from high concentrations of oxygen (oxygen concentration should not exceed 40%) with the possible results of retrolental fibroplasia and blindness. (Retrolental fibroplasia is the formation of fibrous tissue behind the lens of the eye.)

(5) The psychological effects on a patient who is surrounded with the barrier of an oxygen tent. Consider his feelings of:
   (a) Claustrophobia;
   (b) Isolation;
   (c) Limitation to his means of communicating with those around him.

The patient with a tracheostomy

During the course of their work radiographers encounter patients who have had tracheostomies. A tracheostomy is a surgical procedure in which a rounded opening is made in the upper trachea just below the cricoid and thyroid cartilages which enclose the vocal cords. Through this hole in the trachea a tube (known as a tracheostomy tube) is passed, keeping the hole open and giving an airway and access to the patient's trachea, bypassing his nose, mouth and pharynx.

The procedure achieves the following:

(1) It overcomes (through bypassing) any obstruction in the air passages above the tracheostomy opening (i.e. in the mouth, the oropharynx and the larynx);

(2) It allows secretions to be readily removed from the trachea and bronchi by suction (in a patient who cannot cough effectively);

(3) It improves effective ventilation of the lungs;

(4) It facilitates mechanically assisted respiration and it is positively indicated as a procedure to be carried out for any patient who is to have prolonged intermittent positive pressure ventilation (IPPV);

(5) It prevents (by separating the larynx and the pharynx) the inhalation of

food, fluid and secretions by a patient who has paralysis of the muscles involved in swallowing.

Tracheostomy is performed on increasing numbers of patients as a planned procedure in the management of various disorders. It is used in treating (1) patients who have ventilatory failure; (2) patients who are comatose; (3) patients who have lost the nervous control of the act of swallowing; and (4) patients who have undergone laryngectomy (surgical removal of the larynx) and in such cases the tracheostomy is permanent. When the tracheostomy is temporary, as the patient's condition improves the tube is removed and the hole in the trachea is allowed to close.

Examples of disorders in which tracheostomy may be used are: crush injuries to the chest when multiple fractures to the ribs and sternum are interfering with the adequate ventilation of the lungs and the patient is to be aided to breathe by means of a mechanical respirator; conditions involving paralysis of muscles in the pharynx and of the respiratory muscles, when mechanical ventilation will be used as in the previous example; fractures of the cervical spine with spinal cord injury paralysing nerve supply to the thorax (here also mechanical ventilation will be used); severe unstable fractures of the mandible which can cause obstruction of the respiratory tract in its upper parts.

It may be concluded from this list that radiographers using mobile equipment in intensive care units are likely to deal with patients who have had tracheostomy and they may also encounter in the X-ray department patients whose tracheostomies are permanent.

The tracheostomy tube

There are different types of tracheostomy tube as follows.

(1) A plain metal tube. There are three components associated with this tube, which is made of silver. First there is an outer tube (see Fig. 9.3) which has a flange at one end to which the neck piece is attached. The neck piece fits across the front of the patient's neck over the tracheostomy opening, the tube lying within the lumen of the trachea, and it carries tapes which are fastened round the patient's neck and keep the tube in place. Secondly there is an inner tube which fits into the outer one and can be changed and cleaned. The third component is a device called an introducer or pilot – basically a blunt-ended rod with the same curvature as the tracheostomy tube. The surgeon undertaking the tracheostomy puts the introducer with the tracheostomy tube over it into the window he has made in the anterior tracheal wall. He removes the introducer when the outer tube is properly in place and then puts the inner tube into the outer one. The purpose of the blunt-ended introducer (which protrudes from

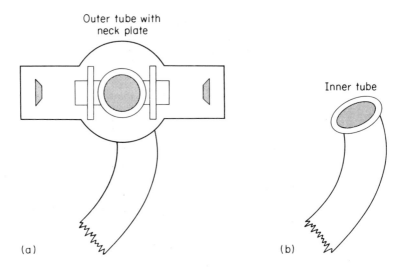

Fig. 9.3 A sketch to show (a) The outer tube of a plain metal tracheostomy tube (the proximal end is shown with its flange and neck plate); (b) the proximal end of an inner tracheostomy tube which fits into the outer tube.

the tracheostomy tube) is to prevent the tube from damaging tissues as it is directed into place.

A silver tracheostomy tube may be fitted with a speaking valve to help the patient whose tracheostomy is permanent.

(2) A plain plastic tube. Three-component plastic tubes are available. Inner tubes make cleaning easy as it can be done without disturbing the outer tube and an introducer makes insertion easier. A plain plastic tube without an inner tube may have an inflatable cuff towards its lower end. Such a tube is sketched in Fig. 9.4. When the tracheostomy tube is in place the cuff lies within the patient's trachea. The cuff can be inflated by means of a syringe attached to the tubing but must also be deflated at regular intervals to prevent tissue necrosis.

When the cuff is inflated as much as is required, the air is prevented from escaping by clamping the tubing between the pilot balloon and the syringe or else by attaching a spigot to the end of the tubing (the end of the tubing is not shown in the figure). The purpose of the pilot balloon is to indicate whether the inflatable cuff (which the operator cannot see as it is inside the patient's trachea) is airtight. The inflatable cuff has two functions to perform. If air, oxygen or an anaesthetic is being pumped into the tracheostomy, all should enter the lungs and none should escape upwards through the larynx. As Fig. 9.5 shows, the inflated cuff can prevent upwards escape as it maintains contact with the walls of the trachea. Secondly the cuff is a barrier to secretions from the upper part of the respiratory tract and prevents their entry to the lower trachea and bronchi.

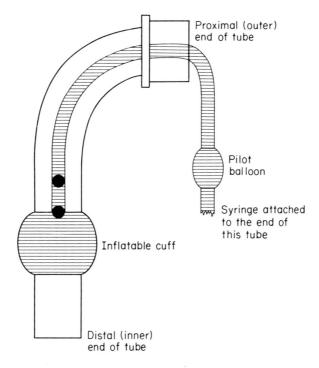

Fig. 9.4 A sketch of a cuffed tracheostomy tube.

Choice of the sort of tracheostomy tube to be used will depend upon why it is being used and what conditions are present in the patient. For a permanent tracheostomy a metal tube is used. If the patient does not need a mechanical ventilator for his respiration and if he can swallow properly and can cough effectively and thus eject any inhaled secretions, then a plain metal or plastic tube (not cuffed) is used. If the patient needs artificial ventilation or is unconscious or is likely to inhale secretions from his mouth or oropharynx, lacking the ability to swallow or a cough reflex, then a cuffed tube is essential so that a barrier may be placed between the upper and the lower parts of the respiratory tract.

The tracheostomy tube is held in place by tapes attached to its neckpiece. The tapes are tied at the side of the patient's neck, where they are less likely to cause discomfort and are more accessible than if they were tied at the back. The tie is by a single bow knot with short loops and long ends. Tapes obviously must not be tied so tight as to constrict the neck but when they are too loose they are dangerous. Loose tapes allow the tracheostomy tube to come out of the lumen of the trachea and yet keep its tip in contact with the tissues immediately in front; here the tube may do a great deal of damage, even to the extent of rupturing the innominate artery.

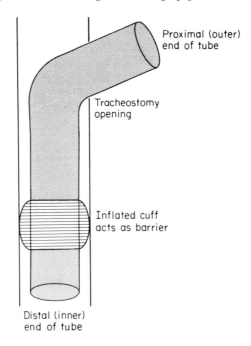

Proximal (outer) end of tube

Tracheostomy opening

Inflated cuff acts as barrier

Distal (inner) end of tube

Fig. 9.5 A sketch to show how the inflated cuff of a cuffed tracheostomy tube fits against the wall of the trachea and acts as a barrier so that gases cannot escape upwards and secretions cannot travel down from above the tracheostomy.

Care of the patient

For a patient who has had a tracheostomy performed proper nursing care of the tracheostomy is extremely important. On it depends the successful treatment of the patient. Where care of the tracheostomy is inadequate, complications such as infection and loss of patent airway often occur. We need hardly say that such complications can kill the patient. Clearly a radiographer does not need to know all the details of caring for a tracheostomy but it may be of help if we indicate important points in the routine care and show what observations a radiographer may usefully make.

Routine nursing care

The routine nursing care of a tracheostomy involves the following procedures.

(1) Caring for the wound.
(2) Ensuring the securing of the tracheostomy tube in its place.
(3) Ensuring the removal of secretions which may block the tube and cause respiratory obstruction.
(4) Ensuring by the use of various devices that the air which the patient

takes in is humidified. This is necessary because the tracheostomy bypasses the upper parts of the respiratory tract in which the air is warmed and humidified in normal breathing. Humidification has an important part to play in keeping secretions fluid; they are then less likely to crust and block the tracheostomy tube.

(5) Changing the tracheostomy tube to prevent the formation of an increasing layer of dried secretions which will narrow the lumen and lead to respiratory obstruction.

(6) Care of the inflatable cuff of a cuffed tracheostomy tube. This cuff must be inflated to just the right amount. Too little and the cuff will fail to act as a barrier in the way it should; too much is dangerous because the cuff may compress blood vessels and damage tracheal tissue. When correctly inflated the cuff must apply some pressure to the tracheal mucosa and to minimize damage to the tissues the cuff is deflated every so often for a brief period.

(7) Observation of the patient to check:
  (a) Adequacy of airway;
  (b) Colour;
  (c) Respiration and pulse.

(8) Provision of such aids to communication as a notepad and pencil and a bell.

Care by the radiographer
A radiographer dealing with a patient who had a tracheostomy as part of the treatment of ventilatory failure should keep the following points in mind.

(1) The patient cannot speak. Unless the tracheostomy is permanent, this loss of normal phonation is only temporary and the patient regains his voice within a few days of the removal of the tube. (Patients who have a permanent tracheostomy after a laryngectomy can be taught to speak without a larynx by using the mouth, tongue, oesophagus and diaphragm; the speech of such patients may sound nearly normal but may be only a whisper.) The speechless conscious patient must communicate with the radiographer by signs and by writing, and there will probably be pencil and paper at the bedside. The radiographer must be understanding and must unfailingly remember that the patient has *not* lost the use of eyes and ears as well as of vocal cords. The patient may feel that their lack of speech makes them an embarrassing nuisance to their attendants. Nothing must be said or done to increase the patient's sense of frustration, the annoyance about their impediment and the feelings of anxiety and depression which their situation brings.

(2) The outer end of the tracheostomy tube must not be inadvertently occluded. The tube clearly must be maintained as a patent airway for the patient. As soon as it ceases to be patent the patient suffers respiratory obstruction and will die if this is complete and maintained. Partial occlusion is distressing as insufficient air gets through and respiration requires more effort. The patient is very conscious of their dependence on the tracheostomy tube as the means of taking in air and the radiographer should understand their apprehensive attitude towards it.

(3) A radiographer should observe the tracheostomy tube, checking that it has not slipped out of position – as it may do if the securing tapes are too loose. If the tube does come out of position the help of nursing staff must be sought *at once* so that it may be restored to its proper place. The danger that, with the tube removed, the tissues will immediately come together and close the hole in the trachea is present in the first 24 to 48 hours post-operatively. During this period the tube must be replaced or tracheostomy dilators inserted very quickly. After 48 hours there is no danger that the hole will close but it remains important not to delay replacement of the tube because its absence may allow secretions to flow into the trachea eventually causing collapse of the lung.

(4) The patient should be observed for signs of respiratory obstruction. Obstruction which is sudden and complete is very infrequent; it could be caused by flakes of dried secretions which have detached themselves from the wall of the tube and are lying across the lumen. Within seconds the patient is cyanosed. Help must be summoned *at once* so that the obstruction may be relieved.

Respiratory obstruction after tracheostomy is much more likely to occur slowly over days from slight beginning to a more advanced state. The causes of such respiratory obstruction may be that the tube is out of position, or being gradually blocked by secretions, or that a tube of too narrow a diameter has been inserted so that insufficient air is reaching the lungs. It is most important that anyone noticing signs of respiratory obstruction in a patient should report the matter to responsible ward staff so that the patient's condition may be investigated and the situation rectified. The signs to be observed are: pallor or cyanosis; an increased and later irregular pulse rate; greater effort in respiration, possibly with widening of the nostrils; reversed or 'see-saw' respiration in which the chest wall moves inwards (instead of outwards as is normal) on inspiration; restlessness; loss of consciousness or deepening of a comatose state.

(5) It is worth noting the state of the tapes which hold the tracheostomy tube in place. If they seem loose the matter should be reported to ward staff. If they become untied they must be re-tied at once and at no time should the tracheostomy tube be left entirely free. The common error is to tie them too loosely. In connection with tying the tapes, it is to be remembered that when the neck is flexed its diameter is less than when the neck is extended. So tapes which are tight when the neck is bent forward will be tighter still when the neck is extended with the head back; and tapes which are loose with the neck extended and the head bent back will be looser still with the neck flexed. It is usual to tie the tapes with the neck flexed to avoid the situation of their being too loose.

The use of suction

In some patients it is necessary to remove the secretions of the trachea and the bronchial tree by a mechanical method that applies suction; this draws the secretions upwards through a catheter. A suction machine is usually electrically operated from a wall socket. Equipment is available which is independent of a mains supply, being operated by a foot pedal, and is thus suitable for taking to the scene of an accident.

A patient who cannot effectively cough up his own secretions requires suction. There may be various reasons why the patient is unable to clear the secretions from his airways:

(1) He may be unconscious.
(2) He may be debilitated;
(3) He may have a depressed cough reflex as an effect of certain drugs;
(4) He may have disabilities such as fractured ribs or muscle paralysis which limit coughing power;
(5) The secretions may be copious, viscous and so tenacious that they are difficult to cough up completely and the patient cannot clear the bronchial tree unaided.

If the secretions are left without attempt to remove them they run down into the bronchi. Here they block some region of the respiratory tract and the normal passage of air is halted in that part of the lung which is distal to the block; air neither enters the lungs on inspiration nor leaves it on expiration. If this process occurs on a large scale the patient drowns in his own secretions and death is certain. It is to prevent this that suction is used. It may also be used in emergency resuscitation of a patient to make sure that there is a clear airway.

Catheters for attachment to the suction apparatus are of a soft plastic, are pre-sterilized by the manufacturer and are disposable, a new one being used for each session of suction. They are available with different diameters. One end of the catheter – the proximal end – is attached to the suction apparatus which is to draw up the secretions through the catheter and deposit them in a bottle or jar (usually filled with antiseptic solution) on the apparatus. The other end of the catheter (the distal end) is inserted into the patient's trachea.

The way in may be through the patient's nose or mouth; if through the mouth it may be down an airway which has been inserted or through an endotracheal tube which has been placed in the trachea via the mouth (*endotracheal* means *inside the trachea*). Or entry may be through a tracheostomy tube in an opening made in the upper trachea (see The Patient with a Tracheostomy, earlier in this chapter).

Figure 9.6 is a sketch of one type of suction apparatus. Mounted on the wheeled base is the electrically driven machine which provides the vacuum pressure for suction. Controls on the metal cover make it possible to switch the machine on and off and to vary the vacuum pressure. Also mounted on the base is a glass jar into which the sucker discharges any matter which it brings up. A piece of tubing can be connected to the aperture on the cover of the jar and to the free end of this tubing (not shown in the illustration) the catheter in use is joined. The machine has a tall handle over it so that it may readily be pushed about from place to place.

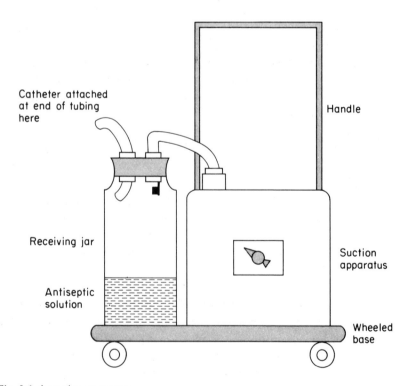

Fig. 9.6 A suction apparatus.

Techniques of using suction

Suction may do a great deal of damage if it is incorrectly applied. Its dangers are threefold:

(1) The introduction of (or the increasing of an existing) infection by the use of techniques which are not sterile, particularly in patients who have had tracheostomy performed recently;
(2) The collapse of part of a lung or the whole lung because suction is continued for too long a time or because a catheter which is too wide is used through a tracheostomy tube;
(3) Damage to the mucous membranes of the tracheal wall by rough introduction of the catheter.

The performance of suction is an important skill for the radiographer to learn as it can be a life-saving one. Patients unable to clear their sections by coughing may require suction, although routine suction of patients is not recommended (Allen, 1988). Noisy or gurgling respirations are a clear indication that suction is required.

The technique is a sterile one as it is important to protect the tracheostomy against infection. The hands must be washed before commencing. A sterile disposable glove is placed on the hand which is to be used for controlling the catheter, keeping the other hand for the 'dirty' work of controlling the suction machine.

The importance of the size of the catheter inserted down a tracheostomy tube is as follows. Once the suction has achieved its purpose of withdrawing sputum (this can be done in a few seconds), continued suction only draws air from the region of the lung where the catheter tip lies. Provided that this air can be easily replaced at once, all will be well (unless suction goes on for a long time), but if the air is not easily replaced, collapse of the lung follows as a serious consequence. Now if the catheter is smaller in diameter than the tracheostomy tube in the trachea (*it should be not more than half the internal diameter of the tube*) air rushes in from outside around the catheter in the tracheostomy tube to replace what is being sucked out and no harm is done. But if the catheter is nearly as wide as the tube, no air can easily get in and the rate of withdrawal can exceed the rate of replacement and trouble follows.

A catheter of sufficient diameter to pass thick mucus is selected but narrow enough to be less than half the diameter of the tracheostomy tube. The distal end is dipped into a sterile lubricating solution and after the solution has been allowed to drain off it, the catheter tip is put into the tracheostomy tube. The catheter is then gently pushed down as far as it will go. The outer end of the catheter is attached to the sucker via a length of sterile plastic tubing and suction can be applied from the apparatus. To lessen the risk of collapsing the lung it is the practice to apply suction only as the catheter is being gradually withdrawn and for no longer than about 3 to 5 seconds.

References

Allen, D. (1988) Making sense of suctioning. *Nursing Times*, 84 (10), 46–7.
Higgins, J. (1990) Pulmonary oxygen toxicity. *Physiotherapy*, 76 (10), 588–92.

Chapter 10
Hysterosalpingography

Hysterosalpingography (uterosalpingography) is the demonstration of the uterine cavity and the uterine tubes by the introduction of a radiological contrast agent. In most cases the purpose of the procedure is to determine whether a tubal obstruction is the cause of sterility. However, evidence is also obtainable of abnormalities of the uterus itself and of its form and position. Anomalies of uterine shape or incompetence of the internal cervical os may be the cause of repeated abortions; so a history of such occurrences is a further indication for hysterosalpingography. Sometimes the examination is undertaken for reasons opposite to those first mentioned, in order to confirm that surgical ligation of the tubes – with the intention of preventing pregnancy – has been successful. Hysterosalpingography usually is conducted under fluoroscopic control by either a radiologist or gynaecologist, or both together.

Preparation of the patient

Hysterosalpingography is not a major procedure. Physically it should not cause undue disturbance and consequently very often is undertaken upon outpatients.

Hysterosalpingography is contra-indicated in certain circumstances:

(1) If the patient is pregnant;
(2) In the presence of acute infection of the genital tract;
(3) During the week preceding and the week following menstruation.

The reasons for the first prohibition are obvious and the risk in the second situation is that of ascending infection. The explanation of the third is that at that point in the menstrual cycle the uterus is very vascular. Introduction of a contrast agent at this stage will lead to *extravasation* into the pelvic cavity.

The timing of the procedure is also important if the possibility of the existence of an early pregnancy is to be avoided.

Ovulation normally occurs halfway through the menstrual cycle and when hysterosalpingography is limited to the period prior to it then the absence of pregnancy can be practically guaranteed. This makes the second week of the cycle the most usual time for the examination but probably not later than the 11th to 15th day after the onset of the previous menstrual period; some extension of the '10-day rule' is permissible, since most of these patients are complaining of infertility. There is some evidence that tubal filling occurs more readily *at* ovulation but routine timing of hysterosalpingography for the day of ovulation would be too inconvenient for many X-ray departments to be practicable. However, it might be appropriate in a special case if an earlier similar investigation had been uncertain in outcome (Chapman & Nakielny, 1993).

It is customary to undertake a pre-arranged number of these examinations during one fluoroscopic session. On the arrival of the patient the radiologist may take a clinical history and will enquire especially into the menstrual history: a period which is irregular in time or of very short duration may suggest the existence of an early pregnancy.

Premedication of the patient is not necessarily indicated and some gynaecologists normally dispense with it. A common cause of pain during the procedure is tubal spasm; factors leading to it may be both physical (arising from the pressure of the injection) and psychological (due to emotional tension in the patient). To avoid these possibilities, some practitioners routinely administer a sedative and anti-spasmodic drug; local anaesthesia of the uterine mucous membrane may or may not be used. In some institutes the practice is to use general anaesthesia, but this requires admission of the patient.

If sedation is customary it will be given to the patient shortly before the procedure is begun. Its use is a matter of clinical opinion and for clinical decision, but where the rule is to employ it, departmental preparations for the procedure obviously must include provision of the appropriate drugs and the means to give them. It should be noted that the form of administration can vary. For example, several drugs may be combined in a *suppository* which is applied an hour before the examination: or a capsule of amyl nitrate may be *inhaled* during the procedure if spasm is seen to occur: sedatives may be given by *mouth or by injection*.

It is of some importance that the bladder be empty during hysterosalpingography because of the close relationship of the uterus to it and the possibility of distorted appearances occurring should it be distended. Every patient should empty her bladder immediately before entering the X-ray room.

The trolley should be prepared in sterile and non-sterile sections, as described elsewhere (see Chapter 4). If several hysterosalpingograms are to be undertaken the trolley must be laid anew for each patient with freshly sterilized instruments and equipment. The following will be required for each patient:

Sterile

- A vaginal speculum (Fig. 10.1).
- A pair of sponge-holding forceps (Fig. 10.2).
- A pair of tissue forceps (Fig. 10.3).
- A pair of vulsellum forceps (Fig. 10.4).
- A uterine sound (Fig. 10.5).
- Dilators, for example, sizes 5 to 8 (Fig. 10.6).
- One 10 ml syringe: this should have finger grips and a screw cap; a bayonet junction or similar non-slip mount for the needle is also useful.

Three types of cannula are encountered commonly.

- The cannula shown in Fig. 10.7 is all metal and the cone near its tip provides a fluid-tight junction at the cervix. Counter-traction on the cervix is needed as the catheter is inserted. To provide such counter-action, Vulsellum forceps are used to grasp the anterior lip of the cervix; patients have described the pain of this manoeuvre as fairly sharp but it should not last longer than a few seconds.
- In another type of cannula, the expanded end is wedge-shaped and has a screw thread. The head of the cannula is screwed into the cervix to provide the necessary fluid-tight joint. No forceps are required in this case; but the instrumentation cannot be said to be free from all discomfort.
- The third variety of cannula is the most elaborate, but the mildest and most comfortable. However, if the patient has experienced a pregnancy and vaginal delivery, there may be scarring of the cervix sufficient to prevent the cannula from fully occluding the external os; and the examination is then impossible to conduct by this means.

  The cannula is described as a suction cannula or a vacuum cannula. Its rounded, acorn shaped plug is made of rubber and is contained within a glass cup which fits over the cervix and is held there by suction. The cannula's operation is associated with a small, hand-operated vacuum pump. This has a pressure gauge to record the degree of partial vacuum created and a screw valve to release the vacuum: it is the vacuum of course which exerts traction on the cervix by means of suction.
- Two small dressing bowls, one to receive sterile swabs and the other for cleansing lotion.
- Two sterile towels and a supply of swabs. A pair of sterile rubber gloves of appropriate size.

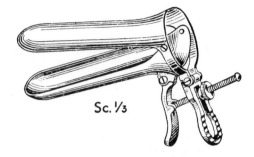

Fig. 10.1 Vaginal speculum. *(Reproduced by courtesy of Charles F. Thackeray Ltd.)*

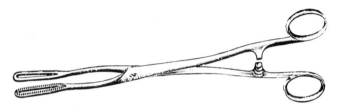

Fig. 10.2 Sponge-holding forceps. *(Reproduced by courtesy of the Genito-Urinary Manu-facturing Co Ltd.)*

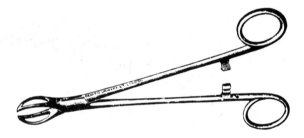

Fig. 10.3 Tissue forceps. *(Reproduced by courtesy of the Genito-Urinary Manufacturing Co Ltd.)*

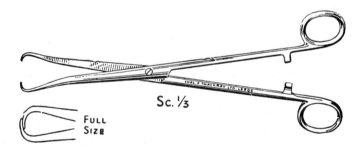

Fig. 10.4 Vulsellum forceps. *(Reproduced by courtesy of Charles F. Thackeray Ltd.)*

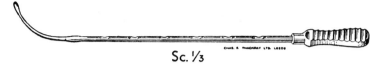

Sc. ⅓

Fig. 10.5 Uterine sound. *(Reproduced by courtesy of Charles F. Thackeray Ltd.)*

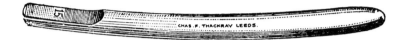

Fig. 10.6 Uterine dilator. *(Reproduced by courtesy of Charles F. Thackeray Ltd.)*

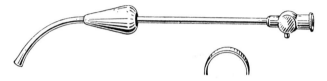

Fig. 10.7 Uterine cannula. *(Reproduced by courtesy of Charles F. Thackeray Ltd.)*

Non-sterile

- A jar of obstetric cream (for example, 'Hibitane' 1%).
- A cleansing lotion for the outer vaginal area (for example, chlorhexidine gluconate, 0.1% in aqueous solution).
- The contrast agent (for example, 'Conray 280' or 'Hexabrix').
- A small mackintosh sheet, or clinical sheets.
- A box of face masks; the disposable variety are satisfactory.
- Also available should be a good light (for example, a standard 'Angle-poise' lamp) and a bin for soiled swabs.

Care of the patient

It is inherent in the nature of hysterosalpingograpy that generally those referred for it are fit young women; they do not suffer from disabling diseases nor such infirmity as to require much physical assistance in the course of the examination. However, we need to remember that associated with every condition of the body there may be – indeed are – psychological factors which often influence to a marked extent our physical reactions.

With this examination there is often (if the purpose of the investigation is to establish the cause of infertility) a highly charge emotional background. These women are anxious for children: their hopes of pregnancy have not been rewarded, no doubt over a period of several years, and every month must carry for them renewed insistence that time is fruitlessly passing. When eventually they reach the X-ray department their infertility will have become a considerable force in their emotional make-up. Inevitably there is some tension associated with the result of the examination: they are very eager to know that they are 'all right'. In addition to this psychological overlay, many of them are genuinely apprehensive about the procedure itself; they are wondering what is actually going to happen to them and whether it will hurt very much.

It is the experience of many who regularly perform hysterosalpingo-graphy that whatever contrast medium is used its commonest side effect is pain, and that there is remarkably wide variation in the degree and even the type of pain experienced. Apart from the effect of the contrast agent, some patients suffer considerable pain from the necessary passage of instruments into the uterus; while in others the discomfort is so light and so transient as not to receive mention. We are perhaps too late to remedy the emotional build-up; certainly we can allay fear, and this is an end worth achievement if we mitigate for any patient the physical distress which she may experience.

In most instances even fairly severe pain resulting from the examination will have passed off within an hour. The patient should be allowed to lie down for a while and a suitable analgesic may be given, such as two (25 mg) pentazocine hydrochloride tablets ('Fortral'). A cup of tea and a hot water bottle are other simple comforts which will be welcome and probably of some benefit. In the majority of cases no other treatment or drug is necessary, though all these patients should be seen again by the radiologist before leaving the department. Fainting can occur after this examination and the patient should be observed after the examination for signs of this. A sanitary towel should be offered as some spotting of blood may occur per vaginum after the examination. Delayed abdominal pain, which may occur several hours later, and profuse bleeding are potentially much more serious complications and the patient should be considered for admission.

While the fact may have little to do with our responsibilities in caring for the patient, the student perhaps will find interest in knowing that this diagnostic investigation appears from time to time to have a therapeutic value. A significant proportion of women investigated for infertility are found to become pregnant shortly after hysterosalpingography has been performed, perhaps due to the removal of some occlusion of the uterine tubes by the introduction of the contrast agent or possibly to some bac-teriostatic action. Various attempts have been made to clarify the reasons for this phenomenon; but whether or not the causes for it are well understood, it is certainly pleasant for the radiographer to meet some of these patients again at the ante-natal clinic!

Reference

Chapman, S. & Nakielny, R. (1993) *A Guide to Radiological Procedures*, (pages 182–185), 3rd Edn., Ballière Tindall, London.

Further reading

Krysiewicz, S. (1992) Infertility in women; diagnostic evaluation with hysterosalpingography and other imaging techniques. *American Journal of Roentgenology*, 159 (2), 253–61.

Chapter 11
Angiography

To obtain radiographic contrast it is necessary for there to be some difference in opacity to X-rays between the structure it is desired to examine and the tissue surrounding it. The student is already familiar with this principle and is aware of the use of radiological contrast agents to provide the opacity within the organ or structure.

In the systemic circulatory system blood vessels are not normally demonstrated on a plain radiograph, because their ability to absorb X-rays is similar to that of the tissues which enclose them. We may detect radiographically the course of a blood vessel in certain instances.

(1) When there are deposits of calcium within its walls. This is an expected finding in many elderly subjects. Radiographs of the pelvis, abdomen, or lower leg, taken for reasons unrelated to any circulatory troubles, quite frequently demonstrate some part of the iliac arteries, the abdominal aorta, or the arteries of the leg, owing to calcific deposits within them.

(2) When a suitable radiological contrast agent has been introduced in sufficient concentration to render the lumina of a group of vessels temporarily opaque in relation to their surroundings.

(3) We may note as a third instance the special case of the vessels in the pulmonary circulation. Since the lungs normally contain air they are more radiolucent than other tissue and provide a natural radiographic contrast. The vessels supplying them appear dense by comparison and are visible on a plain radiograph. It is in fact these vessels which constitute the major part of the pattern of the lung fields radiologically.

However, there is a significant difference between the pulmonary vessels (and cardiac shadow) as they are seen on a plain radiograph, and their visualization following the introduction of a radiopaque contrast agent (as in '2) above). In the first instance we are seeing the external contours of the vessels (or in the case of the heart, the profile of the cardiac chambers). In the second, a contrast medium is present within a vessel or cavity: we see revealed its *internal* outlines and consequently the information obtained is in a different category. The procedures are complementary, and in certain conditions both plain radiographs and contrast agent studies may be necessary for diagnosis.

An examination which entails the introduction of a radiological contrast agent to the circulatory system is loosely described as *angiography*; but radiographers involved with these procedures need and use more informative terms.

Thus, cerebral angiography refers to a contrast examination of the blood vessels of the brain; cardiac angiography (or angiocardiography) to the chambers and circulation of the heart; pelvic venography to the pelvic veins; and peripheral angiography to the arteries of the limbs. Even within these terms there are numerous specific subdivisions which the reader is likely to encounter. For example, brachial arteriography allows the artery of the forearm to be visualized; selective renal arteriography is concerned particularly with the condition of the renal artery; and inferior vena cavography demonstrates the inferior vena cava.

No arteriographic examination is technically simple: all share two significant problems.

(1) **A relatively large quantity of contrast agent (10 to 50 ml) must be introduced** *quickly* **into the vessels under examination**, so as to create an appreciate concentration of radiopaque blood within them. Injection of the contrast agent in a thin, gradual stream – as occurs in the usual form of intravenous injection – fails altogether to fill the lumen of the vessel which is penetrated and is therefore useless in demonstrating any pathology.

    The medium, while appearing fluid in solution, has in fact enough viscosity to offer resistance in the syringe. It is relatively difficult to introduce in sufficient volume and at sufficient speed by hand alone. Some means of manipulating the plunger mechanically at higher pressures is employed in examinations relating to the larger vessels.

(2) **Films must be** *rapidly* **exposed to visualize the filled vessels.** In the large arteries particularly the rate of blood flow is considerable: it approximates to 50 cm per second. The time required for the complete circuit from the heart to the heart again is less than half a minute. To obtain radiographs demonstrating in sequence phases of the blood flow through a group of vessels, films must be changed successively within seconds – or less – of each other: for example, during angiography of the abdominal aorta and its branches, the arterial phase of filling persists literally only for 1 to 2 seconds following injection.

    An automatic changer or more commonly now a device such as a 100 mm cut film camera is necessary, since the series of films cannot be manoeuvred conventionally by hand with sufficient rapidity. Associated with this, the switching of the X-ray unit must be of a type which allows making and breaking of electrical circuits at high rates of repetition – again no mean technical achievement.

The methods available by which these technical difficulties may be met are not our present concern. However, some appreciation of the problem is necessary if the student is to understand that angiography in any form is a complex procedure, requiring careful preparation. It is in fact fundamental to the success of this work that the examining radiologist has a practised team upon whom he can rely and that each should recognize his own personal responsibility for its effective outcome. Even a momentary failure in co-operation, a brief carelessness on anyone's part, can result in the necessity to repeat an entire examination. This not only is an unwarranted addition to the department's work, but carries for the patient – if young especially – certain risks inherent in increased radiation dosage, and the danger of heavy administration of a radiopaque agent containing iodine. The responsibility of repeating such an examination is consequently not light, and it should never become necessary because of some trivial error in procedure.

Preparation of the patient

Angiography is not as a rule undertaken upon outpatients; admission for at least 24 hours is generally advisable to ensure satisfactory preparation and adequate after-care.

Preparation will vary depending on a number of factors.

(1) Whether or not the examination is to be made under a local anaesthetic or, less commonly now, a general anaesthetic.
(2) The preference for a particular premedication of the responsible anaesthetist in the first instance, or in the second of the radiologist who will perform the examination.
(3) The type of vascular study to be undertaken including whether any interventional procedure is likely to form part of the examination.

Within the scope of the present work only the most general observations can be made. However, it is hoped to give the student some indication of the lines which preparation of the patient for these examinations are likely to follow, and so assist in familiarization with a particular departmental practice in any case.

General preparation for abdominal X-ray examination

General preparation is advisable if angiography of the abdominal vessels is to be performed: for example *renal aortography* or *arteriography*. The subject of general preparation has been fully discussed in Chapter 5 and scarcely requires reiteration here. The importance of obtaining adequate bowel clearance with at the same time an avoidance of strong purging may again be usefully noted.

General anaesthesia

General anaesthesia is very rarely required now, but radiographers still need to be aware of the procedure.

Medical and nursing staff will be aware of the usual measures in patient care prior to taking a general anaesthetic. These include:

(1) Possibly an examination of the chest and urine;
(2) The obtaining of written consent to the administration of an anaesthetic;
(3) The removal of make-up from women patients, since artificial colouring on the face and nails might prevent the detection of cyanosis during anaesthesia;
(4) The removal of any denture and jewellery, including a watch. Prior to the procedure some restriction of diet is necessary. Nothing should be taken by mouth for at least 4 hours previously, or longer if the anaesthetist so orders. A heavy meal of any kind must be avoided.

Thirty minutes before the examination the patient will receive the appropriate premedication which the anaesthetist will order. This will be given by hypodermic injection. The trip to the X-ray department must be made on a stretcher or in a bed. The patient should be suitably dressed in an operating gown and comfortably covered with blankets.

During the course of the procedure, the trolley or bed upon which the patient was brought should remain at hand in the X-ray department, to facilitate his removal and return to the ward as soon as possible afterwards. These indeed should be general rules of patient care during any major radiological procedure of this kind, whether or not general anaesthesia is employed. Care of the anaesthetized patient is considered in more depth at the end of this chapter.

Local anaesthesia

The majority of vascular radiological examinations (including many complex interventional procedures) are carried out under local anaesthetic, which may be complemented by some degree of sedation of the patient.

In certain instances general anaesthesia is indisputably indicated.

(1) In the case of children of about 10–14 years of age (babies shortly after birth may be best examined under local anaesthesia).
(2) For a patient unable from any cause to understand what is happening to him and to give reasonable cooperation.
(3) Procedures which require a high degree of co-operation and forbearance from the patient.

When the procedure is to be done under a local anaesthetic the significant feature is to secure, where necessary, adequate tranquillity of the subject by sufficient premedication. Upon the introduction of the contrast agent the patient will experience local warmth and discomfort, even perhaps pain: for example, in the eye, throat and head during cerebral angiography, or in the abdominal region during aortography.

The choice of drugs to induce this happy condition of indifference is a matter for medical decision and is the concern of the radiologist who is to perform the examination. Typical of such premedication is the administration of 10 mg diazepam ('Valium') and 0.6 mg atropine, given by intramuscular injection one hour before angiography.

The patient will normally be admitted to the hospital to allow for preparation beforehand and observations after the procedure. The radiologist will therefore visit the patient on the ward before the examination to explain the procedure and obtain a signed consent form. At the same time the radiologist will examine the patient with particular reference to blood pressure and peripheral pulses (Chapman & Nakielny, 1993). The availability of femoral pulses, for example, will determine the route of introduction of the contrast agent. If a sedative seems to be indicated, the radiologist will arrange with the ward staff for its administration at this time. Some vascular examinations are now conducted on a day case basis with the examination carried out in the morning and the patient then allowed to go home in the evening if all observations are satisfactory.

Preparation of the skin

Preparation of the skin prior to surgery is often stringent. The introduction of an arterial catheter or cannula must be regarded as a surgical procedure, requiring strict observation of asepsis. Some preparation of the skin may be necessary during the time that the patient is on the ward: for example, if the femoral artery is to be punctured in the groin the pubic hair is often shaved. The skin should be washed over a wide area and should be generally clean.

Whether or not any further preparation is undertaken by ward staff, cleansing of the skin with an antiseptic (for example, 'Hibitane' 0.5% in spirit) will be a necessary and immediate preliminary to puncture of the vessel.

The preparation of equipment

The equipment prepared will vary in detail, depending both on the nature of the examination and the technique to be employed. An exhaustive list of what might be required for every angiographic procedure can be of little profit to the student at this stage. In so specialized a subject it is possible here to give only broad guidance, especially with the range of equipment which might be used for associated interventional procedures. What follows is intended rather as general aid than as an absolute statement of what will be done in every department.

In a department undertaking angiographic examination it is likely that a senior radiographer – or a qualified nurse who is seconded to the X-ray staff – will be responsible for the care and organization of the specialized surgical equipment which these investigations require. The time needed for the preparation and disposal of this equipment can be considerable when many such examinations are made.

General statements tend to be vague but we shall have obtained some understanding of the techniques available for angiography – and thus of its required instruments – if we recognize that there are two approaches to the arterial system.

(1) **The vessel concerned may be punctured directly with a needle**. Often this is a percutaneous puncture but in a few instances a small incision of the skin is required to expose an artery (or sometimes a vein). A percutaneous approach is feasible for cerebral angiography through a direct puncture of the carotid artery in the neck; or the aorta may be punctured from behind during translumbar aortography, the needle being introduced on the left side between the rib cage and the bony pelvis. However, direct puncture is now less often undertaken than the procedure described below.

(2) **A catheter may be introduced to a large artery at a point where the vessel passes superficially and may be palpated**. This is followed by such manipulation of the catheter as is necessary to bring its tip within the blood vessel in question.

In many instances the entry of the catheter to the system is made through the femoral artery, which is easily found in the groin with the fingers. The instrument used for the introduction is a special (Seldinger) needle (or an equivalent disposable needle). More accurately, this is a combination of a trocar and cannula, of which the separated parts are shown in Fig. 11.1. When these are fitted together the trocar projects beyond the end of the cannula; it is used to penetrate the anterior wall of the femoral artery through the skin. Arterial blood will flow unmistakably with its characteristic pumping action from the needle, when it is lying within the vessel and

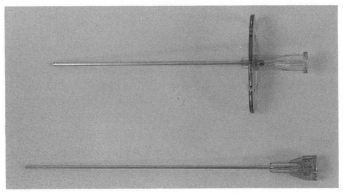

Fig. 11.1 Seldinger trocar and cannula.

on removal of the trocar. With the cannula remaining in position, a long guide wire can be introduced through it to lie within the femoral artery; and is pushed gently along the vessel for a little distance.

Removal of the cannula is easily effected by slipping it off the free end of the guide wire, which is then able to accept the open rounded tip of an intra-arterial catheter. The catheter is gently and steadily pushed along the guide wire, which it needs must follow through the skin puncture; and thus reaches the femoral artery and – from there – can enter the aorta (Chapman & Nakielny, 1993).

Continued advancement and manipulation of the catheter and guide wire together are made to position the catheter correctly for the required examination. For instance, it may remain in the abdominal aorta for bilateral arteriography of the legs; or it may be hooked in the renal artery where this vessel comes off the aorta; or it may enter the cardiac left ventricle; or advance to the vertebral artery in the neck. The progress and eventual position of the catheter are confirmed by image intensifier fluoroscopy as a rule. When all is satisfactory, the guide wire is withdrawn from the catheter, which remains as a channel for the introduction of an appropriate contrast agent.

During angiography surgical asepsis must be maintained. Catheters, needles, syringes and adaptors (taps) are often in a disposable, pre-sterilized category; for example the Seldinger arterial needle depicted in Fig. 11.1. For the reader's guidance we give below a list of the sterile instruments and other accessories which may well constitute a trolley for angiography and can be described as 'basics'. As mentioned previously, the list is indicative only.

Sterile equipment

- 1 angiogram pack (typical contents: 3 towels; 1 ruler; 1 gallipot)
- 3 × 20 ml syringes

- 1 × 2-way tap (see Fig. 11.2)
- 1 × 3-way tap
- 1 × 60 cm connector
- 1 filler
- 2 foil bowls
- 1 scalpel (no. 15 blade)
- 1 Seldinger arterial needle (18G, 2 7/8)
- 1 guide wire
- catheter of a type selected by the radiologist
- 1 vessel dilator
- 1 intravenous giving set
- Gowns and gloves as required.

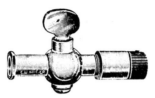

Fig. 11.2 A tap or adaptor for an arterial cannula. *(Reproduced by courtesy of the Genito-Urinary Manufacturing Co Ltd.)*

Drugs and preparations

- 500 ml saline, 0.9%.
- 500 units Heparin.
- A skin cleanser.
- Local anaesthetic (Lignocaine 1% w/v, 5 ml).
- Contrast agent (for instance 'Niopam 300', 1 × 50 ml bottle).

Care of the patient

It should be understood that, in any room where angiography is undertaken, equipment for emergency resuscitation must be readily to hand. During these examinations, particularly if a general anaesthetic is given, perilous situations can arise with great rapidity. It cannot be emphasized too often that the infrequency of trouble must not produce carelessness in providing for it. Minutes spent in fetching some needed items from another room or a distant part of the hospital might be the ones which are to cost the patient their life.

In handling and moving patients for arteriography, certain circumstances may require special attention. For instance, a patient referred for femoral arteriography is likely to suffer from impaired circulation in the lower leg and will be particularly susceptible to injury, even from trivial trauma. Gangrene of the toes, if not actually present in such a case, is a likely eventuality. In manoeuvring such patients in an unconscious condition on the X-ray table, particularly in turning them into the prone position, it is important to provide adequate support for the ankles, so that prolonged pressure on the toes is avoided.

Care in moving the legs is always necessary, and the experienced radiographer in handling these patients should be sufficiently alert to appreciate the possibility of a gangrenous limb, even if coverings on the patient's feet prevent its immediate recognition.

Possible complications of any angiographic procedure are haemorrhage and the formation of haematoma (extravasation of blood into the tissues). This is unlikely to follow a clean arterial puncture, provided adequate compression is applied at the site of penetration following the withdrawal of the catheter or needle. Patience is required here: in some cases it may be necessary to compress the artery for 20 minutes or more before the patient is allowed to leave the department. A firm pressure dressing is applied after the manual compression ceases.

Following his return to the ward, patient observations should be undertaken every 15 minutes for 2 to 3 hours (see below), and the puncture site inspected at the same time for evidence of the development of a haematoma. Less frequent inspections are required for the succeeding 12 to 48 hours. Any of the following signs call for immediate medical attention:

(1) A fall in blood pressure;
(2) A rise in the pulse rate;
(3) Both of these;
(4) Following femoral arterial puncture, pain in the leg and absence of peripheral pulses;
(5) After brachial arteriography, similar occurrences in the arm.

If the examination has been a cerebral angiogram, neurological observations are necessary at 15 minute intervals during the 2 hours which succeed the angiogram.

Patient observations: temperature, pulse, respiration, blood pressure

The taking and recording of the patient's body temperature, rate of respiration, and the rate, force, and rhythm of the pulse beat are basic procedures in medical care. Knowledge of the state of these features in any given patient at a given time provides the doctor with information concerning the condition of the patient, and can give a valuable indication of their general state.

For example, infection gives rise to an increased metabolic rate (this may be defined roughly as the rate at which the body consumes its nutritive fuel), and the increased metabolic rate gives rise to a raised temperature and a faster pulse. Haemorrhage results in a lowered temperature because of the heat loss through loss of fluid, and at the same time the pulse rate increases because the oxygen-carrying capacity of the blood is reduced by blood loss; a low temperature and a rapid pulse may be the first signs given to the doctor that haemorrhage has occurred.

Shallow and slow breathing is found in a state of shock. Laboured and difficult breathing may indicate heart failure. Noisy inspiration is a result of obstruction of the upper air passages.

These are only a few indications of the way in which observation of these features can tell the doctor what is happening in the patient's body, and it is not difficult to see the necessity for meticulously recording them as a part of general nursing care. In the X-ray department the observation of the patient's temperature, pulse, and respiration (sometimes seen abbreviated to TPR) is not required as a routine procedure, and indeed may seldom be done by a radiographer. However, in the event of something untoward happening to the patient while in the department – for example, a patient may collapse or suddenly complain of feeling unwell – it may be necessary to make these observations, and the radiographer should know how they are done. Such observations form a part of the aftercare of examinations such as arteriography.

Temperature

The temperature is usually taken by means of a conventional clinical thermometer, an instrument of which the general features must be familiar to most of us by the time we are old enough to work in hospital. It is made of narrow-bore glass tubing with a wall relatively thick in relation to the bore, and it is filled with mercury. It terminates in a bulb which is the 'business end' of the thermometer, and above this bulb there is a narrowing of the bore so that the mercury level does not fall after the thermometer is taken from the patient.

The normal body temperature remains almost constant in health, although individuals show variation between each other when they are compared. This range of variation is between 35.5°C (96°F) and 37.2°C (99°F), and the average normal temperature is taken as 36.8° C (98.4°F).

The scale of the clinical thermometer is calibrated from 30°C (86°F) to 43°C (109.4°F). With regard to the upper and lower limits, temperatures above about 41°C (105.8°F) and below about 35°C (95°F) are harmful to the life of the body cells, and life cannot long be maintained if the body temperature is a few degrees beyond these upper and lower limits.

It is usual to find the average normal temperature of 36.8°C (98.4°F) marked on the thermometer with a distinguishing point on the scale such as a red line or an arrow head. The thermometer may also be marked with the time it takes to register. It is the usual practice to leave it in place for at least 2 minutes for an accurate record.

It has been the practice to supply in-patients with an individual thermometer for the period of stay in hospital, each thermometer being kept dry in its own container at the patient's bedside. After the patient leaves the hospital, his thermometer and its holder are disinfected by immersion for 30 minutes in an antiseptic solution. They are then stored dry in a clean place. Many wards now use electronic thermometers with disposable covers for each patient.

Before being used, the glass thermometer should be inspected to see that it is in good order and not damaged, and it should then be shaken down so that the mercury is at its lowest level before the thermometer is in contact with the patient. The thermometer is shaken by flicking the wrist to and fro with the thermometer held firmly in the fingers. Care should be taken to see that it is not inadvertently struck against anything during this process. The patient's temperature can be taken in the mouth; or by contact with skin surfaces in the axilla or groin; or by using a special rectal thermometer inserted at the anus.

Taking the temperature in the mouth
It is customary to use the mouth unless there is some reason why it should not be used. It would be contra-indicated if the patient were irresponsible because of their mental state or because they were a young child, if they were unconscious, had a mouth injury or inflammation, if their breathing were difficult or if breathing had to be done through the mouth because of injury to their nose. It should be ascertained that the patient has not recently had any hot or cold drinks.

The bulb end of the thermometer is inserted in the mouth, the patient being instructed to hold the thermometer under their tongue and to keep their lips but not the teeth closed. Needless to say, the patient must not attempt to talk while the temperature is being taken. The thermometer must be read as soon as it is removed, and the reading should be recorded before the mercury is shaken down again.

In ward practice it is usual to keep the record of the patient's temperature and other data on special charts which present the information in the form of graphs, but in the X-ray department the completion of this type of record is not likely to be necessary.

Taking the temperature in the axilla or groin

Since the temperature is being taken in this case by contact between the thermometer and skin surfaces, it is important to see that the contact between the skin and the bulb of the thermometer is well made. This method is therefore not very suitable for extremely thin patients. The skin area should be dried first, and it should be ascertained that the patient has not recently washed the part. If the axilla is being used, the arm is maintained close to the side with forearm flexed across the chest, so that the thermometer is held in the axillary fold. The temperature registered will be $\frac{1}{2}°$ lower than that found in the mouth.

The groin is seldom used except in children, but the same considerations apply as in the use of the axilla.

The pulse

The patient's pulse can be felt at various points in the body where a superficial artery passes over bone, for what is being felt is the expansion of the vessel when the heart chambers contract and pump blood through it. The rate of the pulse beat therefore varies with the rate of the heart, and it will be found normally to be slower in states which slow the heartbeat (for example during rest or sleep), and faster in conditions which increase the rate of the heartbeat (for example during and after vigorous physical exertion).

The usual place for taking the patient's pulse is the wrist, where the artery can be compressed against the palmar aspect of the radius close to the radial styloid process.

For this the patient should be at rest, sitting or lying down, and it is convenient to put the arm into a supported position with the flexed forearm across his chest, palm down. Take hold of the wrist with your opposing hand. The first three fingers of your hand should be firmly applied along the line of the radial artery (palmar aspect of wrist) with your thumb on the dorsal aspect. When you can detect the radial pulse, begin to count the beats, timing with a suitable watch that displays seconds. Unless the rhythm is irregular with the beats unevenly spaced, it is not necessary to count the pulse rate for a full minute. It can be taken for 30 seconds and the figure so obtained is then multiplied by 2 to give the number of beats in a minute.

Once the rate has been determined there are other observations to be made. The radiographer should observe the regularity of the rhythm and its volume (Is it a forceful beat or a weak one?) as these features can be significant. It is also possible to gain an impression of the degree of tension in the artery by testing how easy it is to compress the artery so that the flow is interrupted and the beat stops.

As with the body temperature, the rate of the pulse when the patient is at rest and in health varies little for any one person, although individuals show variation between each other when they are compared. The average normal pulse rate is taken as 72 beats per minute, although rates much slower and much faster than this are considered to be within normal limits for particular individuals. The rate is faster in the newborn (120–140) and in infants, and is slower in old age. Any condition which decreases the metabolic rate slows the pulse rate.

Respiration

The rate of the patient's breathing should be taken without his knowledge. Respiration and the chest movements can to some extent be voluntarily controlled, and once the patient becomes aware that the rate is being counted he may feel self-conscious about it, and it may be difficult to arrive at a true estimate of what the rate is. It is usual to count the respiration with the fingers still on the pulse, and in this way the patient does not know that it is being done. If the patient's hand and arm are laid across his chest with the palm down and the pulse is counted, then the respirations can be noted by the rise and fall of the arm and chest together.

The normal respiration rate is increased by physical exercise and also by emotion. In the average adult at rest the chest rises and falls about 15–20 times per minute. As with the pulse, the rate is quicker in the newborn and in infants. In addition to the rate of respiration, its qualities of depth and regularity are important, and observation should be made of whether the breathing is noisy or quiet.

Blood pressure

The term blood pressure refers to the force exerted by the blood upon the walls of the vessels through which it circulates. This force is related to (1) the force of the heartbeat, (2) the degree of elasticity of the vessel walls, and (3) the amount of blood which is circulating. Various conditions therefore influence the blood pressure.

For example, exercise, emotion, and change of posture from the supine to the erect position all have an effect upon it. As the body ages, hardening of the arterial walls reduces their elasticity so that they offer greater resistance to the blood in circulation; blood pressure therefore rises. A fall in pressure can result from excessive loss of fluid, for example after haemorrhage or severe diarrhoea. Patients in a state of shock also have lowered blood pressure. A maintained rise in blood pressure is called *hypertension*, and a maintained low pressure is called *hypotension*.

When the heart is actively pumping (that is during the systolic phase in the cycle of heart movements), the pressure will support a column of mercury 120 mm high. This figure – 120 mm – is the average systolic pressure, and it is higher than the pressure during the diastolic phase when the heart is relaxed and its chambers are refilling. The average diastolic pressure is about two-thirds of the systolic – that is 80 mm. An expression of the blood pressure usually gives both figures thus: 120/80.

The apparatus which is used to record the blood pressure is known as a sphygmomanometer (Fig. 11.3). This incorporates a mercury gauge on which the pressure in millimetres of mercury will be recorded. In using the apparatus, care must be taken to see that it is so placed in relation to the patient that the latter cannot see the scale of this gauge. There is also a rubber cuff connected to the gauge (the cuff is generally in a cotton cover), and this cuff is fixed evenly round the patient's arm and is inflated with a hand pump to which it is connected. The patient should be reassured as to the ease of the procedure.

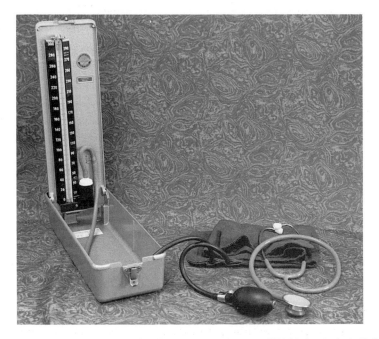

Fig. 11.3 A sphygmomanometer showing mercury column, cuff (folded up), the bulb for its inflation and a stethoscope.

The cuff is put on the patient's arm above the elbow with the centre over the brachial artery. The pulsations of this can be found above the elbow at the medial margin of the biceps by pressure directed posterolaterally. The patient's radial pulse is then located with the finger tips and the cuff is pumped up by compressing the bulb of the pump with the free hand. After a time the pressure that the cuff exerts on the brachial artery is enough to obliterate the radial pulse, its disappearance being detected by your feeling fingers. As the cuff is inflated the column of mercury is seen to ascend the scale: you should note its level when the radial pulse *disappears* and continue to inflate the cuff until the mercury has climbed another 10 mm.

You then place a stethoscope over the brachial pulse above the elbow and slowly release the pressure of the inflated cuff by means of a small threaded screw-valve on the hand-pump. *Note the level of mercury at which is heard (through the stethoscope) the sound as the brachial pulse is re-established:* that level is the **systolic pressure of the blood**. Go on releasing the air and listening to the sound, which *changes to become soft and muffled.* The mercury level at which that change occurs is the **diastolic blood pressure**.

With the blood pressure noted, all the air is released and the cuff of the sphygmomanometer is removed (Pritchard & Mallett, 1992).

The anaesthetized patient

Although there is a reduction in X-ray departments of procedures which involve the use of a general anaesthetic, care of the unconscious patient is still an important part of a radiographer's responsibility. Even though this care is of a temporary character and short duration for any particular patient, lack of knowledge can result in disasters which may occur very quickly. The radiographer must understand the mishaps which are liable to occur, and must know the simple yet important principles of care of such a patient, not only during the period of recovery from anaesthesia but also prior to and in the course of its induction.

Anaesthetics

Anaesthesia is loss of sensation, particularly those of touch and pain: there may or may not be accompanying loss of consciousness. Anaesthesia may come about as an abnormality in a process of disease but in the present context we are of course considering only its deliberate induction by medical hands using anaesthetic agents to cause it. These agents are in two classes as follows.

(1) **Local anaesthetics** which, by acting on nerves and nerve tracts, affect local areas only and leave the patient conscious. Examples are procaine; lignocaine; EMLA cream.
(2) **General anaesthetics** which affect the entire body and result in loss of consciousness when the agent acts on the brain. Examples are vapours and gases such as ether, nitrous oxide, methyoxygluorane; agents for intravenous injection such as sodium pentothal.

Before surgical procedures and general anaesthetics, the patient is prepared by the administration of certain drugs. This preparation is called pre-medication and the objectives are as follows:

(1) **To allay anxiety and induce drowsiness** with agents such as morphine, pethidine, the barbiturates;
(2) **To diminish salivary and bronchial secretions** with agents such as atropine, hyoscine;
(3) **To inhibit the parasympathetic nerve supply** and thus restrain cardiac arrhythmias (atropine, hyoscine as before);
(4) **To give analgesia and sedation** for the immediately post-operative period;
(5) **To ease the induction and maintenance of anaesthesia**.

Before anaesthesia

A patient who comes to the X-ray department for any radiological procedure which requires the administration of an anaesthetic, either local or general, will often be already under sedation by the time the radiographer receives them.

No sedated patients should be left alone at any time in the X-ray department unless in a bed with cot sides. The patient will arrive in the X-ray room in the company of a nurse but it is quite probable that the latter must then leave to return to her duties on the ward. The radiographer who receives the patient should observe the following procedure.

(1) Greet the patient by name, giving them also some words of comfort and confidence. This is an important part of psychological care. Vascular examinations in particular can be traumatic and our suites of equipment look daunting.
(2) Check carefully the patient's identity, referring to the case notes, the patient's hospital number, the X-ray requisition form and any previous radiographs.
(3) Check with the nurse, the case notes and personal observation that the patient has been prepared for the procedure, particularly that any denture normally worn has been removed.
(4) If the patient has to wait on the X-ray table make them as comfortable as possible.
(5) Be quiet. If others are in the room, unnecessary noise and conversation should be avoided, as such stimuli may excite or confuse the patient.
(6) If the patient wishes to talk, reply gently, briefly and reassuringly.
(7) Remain with the patient. And do not struggle with a patient who becomes restless, either at this time or during induction of general anaesthesia. Assistance should be obtained when necessary.

During induction of general anaesthesia, the anaesthetist is likely to require help from a member of the radiographic staff if a nurse is not available for this purpose. At this time conversation should be avoided as far as possible. If words are necessary they must be carefully chosen: as consciousness fades so hearing becomes more acute and a patient can be easily alarmed and upset by comments which may not be properly understood.

A number of ways of producing anaesthesia are available but their discussion is irrelevant to the purpose of this book. In the X-ray department the probable method will be by inhalation of gases, preceded by the intravenous injection of a rapidly acting agent. Several stages of anaesthesia are described below and are shown in Table 11.1.

Table 11.1 Stages of general anaesthesia.

Stage I	*Stage II*	*Stage III*
Initial excitement; limbs and eyes move; pupils dilate; muscle spasm.	Loss of voluntary control of nervous system.	Entire relaxation. No muscle rigidity. Deep regular breathing Sluggish corneal reflex.
Nervous system at first remains under voluntary control.	Brisk corneal reflex.	
Loss of peripheral sensation. Swallowing movements. Brisk corneal reflex.		

Note. The corneal reflex is the response of the eye to irritation of the cornea. If a light touch is made on the cornea of the eye, the eyelids instantly close or try to close. This reflex is lost only in deep anaesthesia or coma.

(1) **Analgesia.** The nervous system remains under control but the patient loses peripheral sensation. During this stage he may make swallowing movements.
(2) **Excitement**, which may be observed in movements of the limbs and eyeballs, dilatation of the pupils and muscle spasm. The purpose of administering the short-acting anaesthetic is to avoid this stage. The patient usually falls rapidly and easily asleep.
(3) **Surgical anaesthesia** which will be moderate or deep depending upon the requirements of the operation or procedure; in the X-ray department only light or moderate anaesthesia should be required.

In attending the anaesthetist the radiographer's function may include the following:

(1) Assisting with any intravenous injection;
(2) Handing to the anaesthetist any instruments, drugs or apparatus they may need;
(3) Under the anaesthetist's direction, adjusting the flow of a transfusion, or checking the pulse or blood pressure of the patient.

At no stage of the procedure should the anaesthetist be left wholly alone with the patient, particularly during either induction or termination of the anaesthetic. Emergencies may occur which are difficult for one person to handle without assistance of some kind. From another point of view, if the patient is a woman a male anaesthetist should have a chaperone present as a safeguard against hallucinatory allegations of unprofessional conduct towards her.

Following general anaesthesia

Care of the unconscious patient should follow the same rules, whether their condition has resulted from anaesthesia or another cause. The patient must never be left alone while they are in the X-ray department but must be kept under observation. In the case of the anaesthetized patient the anaesthetist will terminate anaesthesia gradually and will indicate when the patient is fit to be moved from the table and return to the ward.

In placing an unconscious patient either on the X-ray table or on a trolley it is important to see that their arms are not in such a position that they will be lying on them when they are laid down. Nor should the patient's arms be allowed to dangle over the edges of the trolley or table and hang down towards the floor.

The commonest cause of death in the anaesthetized patient has been said to be obstruction of the airway produced by the relaxed tongue falling against the posterior wall of the pharynx; the patient is unable to breathe by reason of this obstruction. It is important, therefore, to see that a clear airway is maintained, and this is the first essential in looking after such a patient. In some cases a rubber airway may have been inserted, and there is then less likelihood of obstruction occurring. However, if the patient is restless and tries to eject the airway, it is better removed.

If the patient has to lie supine, his lower jaw should be held forward. This is done by pulling the jaw forward so that the lower teeth are beyond the upper ones. This keeps the tongue forward and the airway clear. If there is risk of the patient vomiting, the head should be turned to one side.

The vomiting patient is in danger of inhaling vomit. In the X-ray department this risk can be removed if the patient is put on a tilting table and tipped a few degrees head downwards. A tilting table is the best one for an unconscious patient. If this is not available, the head should be turned to one side and the shoulders tilted sideways so that the head is really well turned. It should be ascertained that the airway is clear.

An advantageous position for the patient is one giving postural drainage. That is a semi-prone position, halfway between lying on one's side and lying face downwards (Fig. 11.4). The arm of the side on which the patient is lying should be placed behind them (*not* underneath the patient). The head is turned on one side with the face rotated slightly downwards.

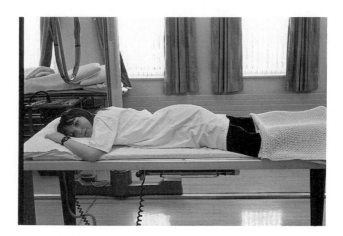

Fig. 11.4 The semi-prone recovery position.

The patient's colour should be observed for cyanosis. The term cyanosis means that the patient is beginning to turn blue, and this will be observed in the face. It is a sign that the blood is lacking in oxygen. The blueness will show first in the tips of the ears and the nose, and immediate action should be taken. It should be made certain that the airway is clear, oxygen should be given by mask and medical advice sought.

If the patient stops breathing a method of artificial respiration which can be instantly and easily applied is one which is called expired air resuscitation (see pages 235–7).

It is to be emphasized that these considerations in the care of the unconscious patient – the importance of seeing that a clear airway is maintained and that the patient can vomit in safety – apply whatever may be the reason for the patient's unconsciousness, whether it is due to anaesthesia or other causes. If the student radiographer is left alone with an unconscious patient and a change in the patient's condition is detected (for example, they become cyanosed or stop breathing), the student should *not* run out of the room to fetch the assistance of seniors, leaving the patient alone. Instead the attention of others should be attracted by calling, and such procedures as seem immediately helpful should be initiated without delay. Some departments now have panic buttons available for such circumstances.

If the patient is not completely unconscious but is semi-conscious, nothing should be given by mouth.

References

Chapman, S. & Nakielny, R. (1993) *A guide to Radiological Procedures*, (pages 201–206), 3rd Edn., Baillière Tindall, London.

Pritchard, A.P. & Mallett, J. (1992) *Manual of Clinical Nursing Procedures*, (pages 318–341), 3rd Edn., Blackwell Science, Oxford.

Chapter 12
The Spinal Column

Myelography/radiculography

The terms *myelography* and *radiculography* are applied to the subarachnoid injection of a radiological contrast agent for the purpose of examining the spinal cord and neighbouring structures. Such a procedure will demonstrate, for instance, the site of a prolapsed intervertebral disc which is causing pain through interference with nerve roots.

The first radiological contrast agent in general use for examination of the spinal cord was an oil-based iodine compound ('*Myodil*'). The substance remained in the spinal column for many years and has been found to have harmful after-effects which are now the subject of litigation. This has been succeeded by non-ionic water-soluble agents such as iopamidol ('*Niopam*') and iohexol ('*Omnipaque*'). When one of these is injected through lumbar puncture, the lumber nerve roots and sheaths are particularly demonstrated and the name *lumbar radiculography* is used to describe the procedure. When the examination includes the thoracic and cervical regions of the cord, the term *myelography* is applicable.

Whichever part of the cord is under investigation, the contrast agent is introduced most often by *lumbar puncture*. Its flow along the subarachnoid channel is then controlled by fluoroscopy on a tilting table; if it is to be fully suitable for cervical myelography such a table should provide 90° Trendelenburg tilt, to enable the contrast agent to flow readily from the patient's lower back to his neck. Occasionally for a cervical myelogram, the contrast agent is introduced directly in the neck by a suboccipital lateral puncture at the level of C1/C2. Because this is the more hazardous approach, direct cervical puncture is performed more usually by a specialist neuroradiologist than in the majority of general radiodiagnostic departments.

The practices of radiculography and myelography require strict asepsis, since the introduction of any infection may result in meningitis; this is a serious illness. Injection of the contrast agent is made usually in the radiodiagnostic room by the supervising radiologist; it immediately foreruns fluoroscopy, accompanied by such exposure of radiographs as is necessary to record the region examined and as the fluoroscopic inspection may indicate. The selected X-ray room should be prepared beforehand so that it can be regarded as 'clean'. It would be unacceptable practice if a radiographer, for instance, allowed the X-ray table to proceed immediately from a barium enema examination to a myelogram without a thorough cleansing of its surface and adjacent parts; the use of a bactericidal spray is appropriate.

Preparation of the patient

Myelography is not an examination to be performed on outpatients. Usually it is one of several investigations which have to be made to obtain the diagnosis of a spinal lesion and these require admission to hospital for a period. Consequently, it is the immediate responsibility of nursing staff to prepare the patient; but manifestly there is an equal charge on the X-ray department to ensure that the ward sister knows of the radiologist's requirements in this respect, and that the patient receives full and correct information about this invasive procedure (Foote, 1991; Flemming, 1994).

Depending on the patient's condition, preparation may include tranquillization, but the general practice is not to use any premedication. Patients must be well hydrated for radiculography/myelography and to encourage this should eat and drink normally beforehand; a light meal is allowed on the morning of the examination. The following are significant points in a patient's preparation:

(1) Obtaining his informed consent to the examination;
(2) Ample hydration and normal diet whenever possible;
(3) Removal of jewellery and any denture;
(4) Clothing (a theatre gown open at the back, pants, socks);
(5) Transport to the X-ray department in his bed.

Preparation of the trolley

A trolley for radiculography/myelography should be prepared in upper (sterile) and lower sections in accordance with usual practice. The following is a typical preparation.

Sterile

- 2 gallipots.
- 1 × 10 ml syringe.
- 1 × 5 ml syringe.
- Needles: typically 1 × 21G, 1 × 23G.
- A filler.
- A lumbar puncture needle, 22G. (Two examples are seen in Fig. 12.1.)

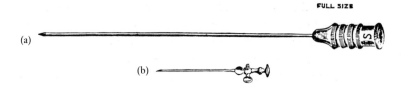

Fig. 12.1 Lumbar puncture needles. (a) Harris type (b) Greenfield pattern. *(Reproduced by courtesy of Down Bros. and Mayer & Phelp Ltd.)*

- A connector. (This is a length of about 200 mm of tubing fitted with adaptors which enable it to make a link between a syringe and the lumbar puncture needle *in situ*; it allows manipulation of a loaded syringe with no disturbance of the needle's position.)
- An absorbent towel for draping the patient; this should have a central longitudinal cut-out for exposure of the lumbar region of the spine, whilst covering the remainder of the trunk.
- A pair of rubber gloves of appropriate size.
- Gauze swabs.

Non-sterile

- A local anaesthetic, such as Lignocaine.
- The contrast agent; for example, 'Omnipaque 180 mg 1/ml' in 10 ml ampoules (10–15 ml being the usual dose for radiculography/myelography).
- A skin cleanser, such as 'Hibitane' 0.5% in spirit.
- 2 specimen bottles (for collection of cerebrospinal fluid for subsequent laboratory analysis).
- A disposable razor (for depilation of the lumbar region if it proves necessary).
- Some small adhesive plasters for sealing of the needle wound.

Care of the patient

No patient who has undergone radiculography/myelography will describe it as an enjoyable procedure. Many subjects have suffered pain from the condition under investigation. Since many movements of the body involve the spinal column, the patient may be able to do little that does not aggravate their distress.

A patient referred for radiculography/myelography is rarely a stranger to the X-ray department; plain radiographs of the spine will have been taken, perhaps on several occasions, before the decision to proceed to a contrast examination is made. Even so, a degree of familiarity with the surroundings provides little comfort and a patient should be reassured that it is the intention to make investigation as easy as possible. This encouragement should include an explanation of what is to follow.

A patient should be warned that they will be required to lie prone for some while and that they may be tilted head downwards or heels downwards at various times. The patient should be shown the shoulder supports and handgrips and any harness or other support to be used; and should be instructed in their application. It is important to give sustained reassurance to patients that they will not be allowed to fall, no matter in what way it may be necessary to tilt them. Expressions of encouragement and timely indications that all is proceeding well help a patient the better to endure a trying investigation.

The radiographer who fits a harness or other myelographic attachment to the X-ray table, prior to the examination, is responsible for seeing that such auxiliaries are correctly in place and are in good order. Serious accidents have occurred because of their faulty use. During the procedure, attention must be given immediately to a patient who says that they are slipping or insecure.

It is understood that the X-ray room will have been fully prepared before the patient's arrival. As far as possible, other examinations should be scheduled to avoid any overlap, so that sufficient time may be given to adequate organization of technical equipment and the patient kept waiting as little as possible, either to enter the room or while various needed items are made ready. This is a good practice in respect of any major radiological procedure.

The contrast agent is introduced via a **lumbar puncture** into the subarachnoid space. The spinal cord terminates below the first lumbar vertebrae and thus the site for lumbar puncture is commonly betweer the fourth and fifth lumbar vertebrae. Radiologists have personal preferences as to the position of the patient for the introduction of the needle but commonly they are asked to lie on their left side on the table and to flex the knees up to the chest. This widens the intervertebral spaces and makes the needle easier to insert (Allen, 1989). The area is infiltrated with local anaesthetic and then the lumbar puncture needle is inserted. A small sample of cerebrospinal fluid is removed and sent for laboratory analysis prior to injection of the contrast agent (see Figs. 12.2 and 12.3).

Although those now in use are less toxic than earlier media, it is usual during radiculography/myelography to try to avoid an entry of the contrast medium to the cranium. Such intracranial spill may produce irritation of the cortex and is considered to influence significantly the severity of the examination's side effects.

A secondary consideration is the radiographic disability when contrast agent is 'lost' in the skull (being difficult to recover from the cranium to the

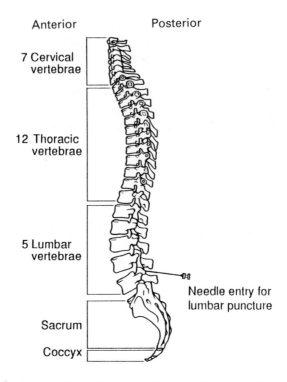

Anterior   Posterior

7 Cervical
vertebrae

12 Thoracic
vertebrae

5 Lumbar
vertebrae

Needle entry for
lumbar puncture

Sacrum

Coccyx

Figure 12.2 Lateral view of spinal column to show needle entry site for lumbar puncture. *(Reproduced by courtesy of the Medical Art Department, The Royal Marsden NHS Trust.)*

spinal portion of the subarachnoid space); the remainder may be insufficient in quantity for satisfactory imaging and thus spoil the examination.

Movement of a recumbent patient during and immediately after radiculography/myelography should be managed carefully, in order to inhibit intracranial spill of the contrast agent. In the prone position the patient should be asked to keep their neck slightly extended, and if necessary should be helped to do so. When a patient must lie thus for some time, the head should be turned sideways and adequate support with firm pillows provided for the cheek; if only one pillow is available, it is often advantageous to fold this double. During any turning of the patient to the lateral decubitus, the head can usually be kept at a higher level than the body by an assistant, who should apply gentle lateral flexion to the neck in the appropriate upward direction. During cervical myelography when a prone patient must lie looking straight ahead, a firm support beneath the chin should maintain extension of the neck without much discomfort. Following radiculography/myelography a patient will remain in hospital for a further 24 hours at least and should be encouraged to increase fluid intake during this time. The patient should not drive a car for 48 hours after the examination.

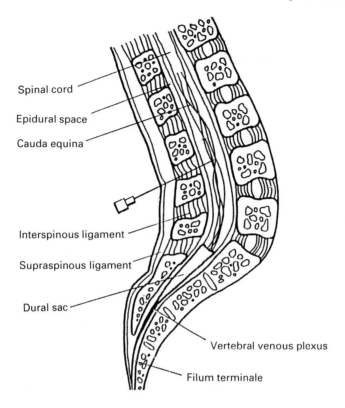

Spinal cord

Epidural space

Cauda equina

Interspinous ligament

Supraspinous ligament

Dural sac

Vertebral venous plexus

Filum terminale

Fig. 12.3 Lumbar puncture. Saggital section through lumbosacral spine. *(Reproduced by courtesy of J. Mallett, The Royal Marsden NHS Trust.)*

Side effects either may be immediate (that is, present at the end of the procedure), or may develop or persist subsequently during several hours. Headache, of varying severity and duration, is the most common complaint; other recognized effects include nausea, vomiting, and infrequently dizziness. Much more serious reactions, embracing mental changes and epileptic seizures, have been known to occur but are now unusual (Bartholomew, 1992).

A patient leaving the department after radiculography/myelography should have the bed's headrest adjusted in order to sit upright. Traditional aftercare of a patient who has had a lumbar puncture entails bed-rest for 12 to 24 hours; nursing staff may be advised to maintain some elevation of the patient's head, either with two pillows or by means of an upward tilt of the bed of about 20 degrees. Some radiologists consider that bed-rest for 24 hours is not required. Unnecessary movement should be avoided, but patients may sit upright in a chair and should be allowed up to visit the lavatory.

Discography

Radiographers should distinguish precisely between radiculography and discography. In the course of discography a selected intervertebral disc is visualized by the introduction of a contrast agent to the nucleus. Such direct investigation of the disc itself may give a definitive diagnosis of its condition, when this is clinically suspect but not radiologically proven by other means. If it is necessary to examine more than one intervertebral disc, each must have a separate injection.

In some cases of prolapsed intervertebral disc – particularly in young subjects – a modification of discography offers an alternative treatment to laminectomy; and is much simpler. For this procedure, following correct placement of a needle in the nucleus, an injection of chymopapain is given and will result in dissolution of the offending disc. When successful, this remedy is an attractive means to cut the Gordian knot of lower back pain (Chapman & Nakielny, 1993).

Needles used for discography are significantly longer than lumbar puncture needles; and an operator needs care and skill to penetrate the nucleus accurately. Television fluoroscopy is essential to establishment of the needle's position and will include horizontal-beam fluoroscopy. This may be provided by an additional image intensifier on a C-arm, if other equipment is not available.

A trolley for discography

Radiographers preparing a radiodiagnostic room for discography may find it convenient to set out two trolleys. One of these – the 'scrub up' trolley – is small and contains the following sterile items: towels; gloves; a gown; a nail brush; and a box of face masks. A larger trolley should be made ready in sterile and non-sterile sections, for which a typical layout is listed below.

Sterile

- 4 towels.
- 4 towel clips.
- Syringes: 10 ml; 5 ml; 2 ml.
- Needles: 2 × 21G, $1\frac{1}{2}$; 1 × 21G (12.5 cm); 1 × 26G (12.5 cm). The 12.5 cm needles are suitable for penetration of the disc nucleus.
- 2 fillers.
- 1 gallipot.
- Swab-holding forceps.
- Gauze swabs.
- Connectors or extension tubes.

Non-sterile

- A skin cleanser, such as 'Hibitane' 0.5%.
- A local anaesthetic, such as Lignocaine 1% (10 ml).
- The contrast agent ('Niopam 200' in 10 ml ampoules).
- Diazepam ('Valium') for injection.
- Hydrocortisone for injection.
- Files for opening ampoules.
- Small adhesive plasters.

References

Allen, D. (1989) Making sense of lumbar puncture. *Nursing Times*, 85 (49), 39–41.

Bartholomew, A. (1992) A study of Iohexol lumbar myelography to identify adverse reactions and evaluate their causes. *Radiography Today*, 58 (661), 21–4.

Chapman, S. & Nakielny, R. (1993) *A Guide to Radiological Procedures*, (pages 372–3, 3rd Edn., Baillière Tindall, London.

Flemming, S. (1994) Increasing patient awareness before, during and after radiculography. *Radiography Today*, 50 (679), 16–20.

Foote, S. (1991) Myelography – an assessment of communication with a view to improving patient care and standardising information. *Radiography Today*, 57 (652), 20–24.

Chapter 13
Complementary Imaging

Introduction

The term X-ray department, although in common usage, is no longer wholly appropriate to the range of diagnostic imaging investigations which are now undertaken. The student radiographer will undertake experience in most complementary imaging modalities and, although it is still recognized that these modalities are ones in which radiographers will undertake additional training after graduation, it remains important for the student to be aware of the principles of patient care in each of the areas of complementary imaging. We shall consider each of the modalities in turn.

Ultrasound

The role of ultrasound as a diagnostic imaging modality is still expanding, partly because of the lack of radiation hazard connected with its use but also because of the portability of the equipment for certain applications. As mentioned at the beginning of Chapter 8, ultrasound has virtually replaced the use of diagnostic radiography for investigations of the biliary system, and this is also happening in other areas of diagnostic imaging.

In our dealings with patients who may attend the ultrasound department it must be remembered that the examinations undertaken tend to fall into two categories: (1) examination of patients who are suspected of suffering from a particular illness, and (2) patients who may be, or wish to become, pregnant. It is important to remember that pregnancy is not an illness. McLellan (1990) points out that the well-woman 'believes she is well but is afraid she may not be' or that her baby may not be. Owing to its very specialized nature, mammographic breast screening has not been specifically dealt with in this volume, but the same principles of patient care apply since these are also well-women.

McLellan points out that well-women may be much more enquiring than sick patients and require careful handling in terms of communication skills. Crawley (1992) in her observations of patient–radiologist interactions in ultrasound, comments extensively on the expectations of patients for a

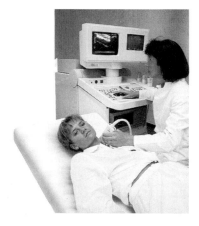

Fig. 13.1 Medical ultrasound. *(Reproduced courtesy of Siemens plc.)*

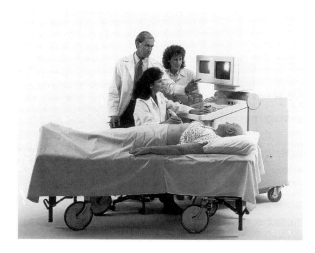

Fig. 13.2 Medical ultrasound – a case conference. *(Reproduced courtesy of Siemens plc.)*

diagnosis and the difficulties of the passing on of bad news. Crawley comments that even when a patient is told that there is nothing abnormal, they may not necessarily be reassured as they may have to face further procedures to find out the cause of their symptoms. A particularly difficult situation arises when there is the appearance of an abnormal fetus on the scan. Increasingly, sonographers are being trained in counselling skills to enable them to communicate sensitively with patients where this occurs.

Preparation of the patient

If the investigation is of an abdominal organ (for example the gall bladder), it is usual to instruct the patient to observe the department's customary preparation for abdominal radiology. This preparation is likely to include:

(1) The taking of an aperient two days before the examination;
(2) Limitation to a light diet, with special avoidance of gas-producing vegetables, on the day preceding the examination.

However, the patient should not be dehydrated and may be asked to drink two glasses of water or orange juice before coming to the X-ray department. Particularly during gynaecological examinations, a full bladder – which naturally is transonic – is an advantageous 'landmark'.

A patient for an abdominal or pelvic scan should undress in accordance with usual practice.

During scanning the use of a coupling medium is always necessary, in order to avoid an air gap between the skin surface and the sonar probe. The coupling medium will be applied by the sonographer before beginning a scan and from time to time as need occurs; it should be to hand with the equipment. The agent most often employed is an aqueous gel which can be easily removed from the skin with a paper towel or tissue; these, too, should be available, together with a bin for their disposal.

Radionuclide imaging

A wide range of radionuclide examinations now exists and preparation protocols tend to differ in each department. The examinations can usually be performed on outpatients. Research is in progress regarding the amount of information which should be given to patients before a radionuclide examination. The approach adopted by most radiographers is to discuss the examination in terms of a 'risk vs benefit' approach. The research appears to show that an outline of the examination is all that patients require, and that any detailed discussion of the risks of the investigation can make them very frightened and can increase the risk of non-compliance. Scan times are still comparatively long – up to 45 minutes in some cases – and it is therefore important to ensure that the patient understands the need to keep very still during the examination. There may be quite a long waiting period between the injection of the radionuclide and the scan itself and arrangements must be made for the patients to be made comfortable somewhere before the scan commences.

It has been stated that there are no after-effects from a radionuclide examination (Bryan, 1987) but patients have been known to experience minor headaches, nausea and dizziness for up to a week after the examination has taken place. Following certain procedures (in particular bone scans) patients are encouraged to drink copious fluids as this encourages the flushing out of the radionuclide via the kidneys and bladder and helps to reduce the radiation dose from the investigation. Parents with children are advised not to have them on their knee for up to 12 hours after the scan owing to the concentration of the radionuclide in the bladder.

Computed tomography

Research has shown that patients need to be informed in advance about the requirements of the examination – in particular the administration of intravenous injections and oral contrast agents which are now commonly used to enhance structures under investigation (Robinson, 1992).

Computed tomography (CT) is no different from other X-ray investigations in the respect that the patient's preparation is governed by the needs of the region to be examined. For instance, in the case of an abdominal scan, preparation of the patient is often similar to that used for a plain radiograph of the kidneys, ureters and bladder: the patient may be asked to avoid green vegetables and follow a light diet for two days; the patient may be given a bowel evacuant on the morning before and on the morning of the CT examination. On the other hand, CT scans of the chest and limbs do not require any special preparation.

The use of contrast agents

The use of a radiological contrast agent to enhance cerebral and abdominal CT images is well established. The practice is effective because the presence of the contrast agent increases differences between the attenuation values of various tissues; and thus improves accuracy in the recognition of tissue change. The contrast agents employed in this application should be from the non-ionic, water-soluble iodinated group which are discussed in Chapter 3 under the heading Iodine Preparations. An appropriate example is 'Omnipaque' (iohexol) in a concentration of 300 mg iodine/ml and a dose of 2 ml per kilogramme of body weight; but it is to be expected that radiological practice is not universal and varies to some degree.

Sometimes the preparation of a patient who is to have an abdominal scan may include the administration of Gastrografin about $1\frac{1}{2}$ hours beforehand: 6 ml of Gastrografin is mixed with 250 ml of water (about half a pint) and is taken by mouth. The effect of the dilute contrast agent is strongly to opacify the gut and thus to facilitate the identification of bowel loops – which might otherwise be confusing – during CT.

The patient may be frightened by the size and appearance of the scanner when entering the scan suite (Ehrlich & McCloskey, 1989 p 225). It is important to explain to the patient what is going to happen during the procedure and that there is an intercom system which will enable the radiographer to be in constant contact during the examination. Research has also shown that patients are surprised (and again may be rather frightened) by the noise made by the scanner (Robinson, 1992). It is important for radiographers to remember that what we take for granted can be very distressing for a patient who is already in an anxious state. The comparative ease of operation of some CT machines does not obviate the need to spend time with the patient in order to ensure a successful outcome.

As with the other scanning procedures the need to keep still must be emphasized and patients should be kept informed of what is happening via the intercom at each stage of the examination.

Magnetic resonance imaging

This comparatively new imaging modality does not use ionizing radiation but achieves images by means of magnetic fields and radiowaves. On the face of it the equipment seems similar to CT scanning, but it is in fact very different. Prior to entering the scanning area (and therefore the magnetic field) both patients and other visitors are asked to fill in questionnaires which ask primarily about whether the respondent has ever had any metal implants; these would include hip replacements, artery clips, heart valve replacements or pacemakers. If there is any possibility that the patient may have sustained any metal fragments in the eye then orbital X-rays are taken prior to the scan (Ehrlich & McCloskey, 1989 p 222). Certain metal implants may be dislodged by the very powerful magnetic fields; others may cause artefacts on the scan image. Items such as hearing aids, pens and other metallic objects and credit cards must also be left outside the scanner suite owing to the high peripheral magnetic fields.

Research has been undertaken into the high levels of patient anxiety which are experienced by those attending for magnetic resonance (O'Connor, 1993; Thorp *et al.*, 1990). A proportion of this anxiety has been associated with the fact that patients may come expecting that the outcome will be that they have cancer (Thorp *et al.*, 1990).

O'Connor (1993) concluded that patients found the equipment very intimidating, but as with the research into radionuclide imaging, would not particularly have welcomed a more detailed explanation beforehand ('I would really have panicked and refused the examination altogether', was one response she received). Claustrophobia can be a big factor in whether or not

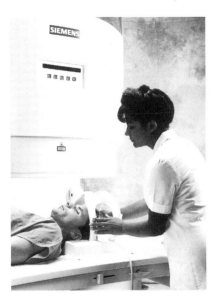

Fig. 13.3 Magnetic resonance imaging using a head coil. *(Reproduced courtesy of Siemens plc.)*

patients go ahead with the examination, and radiographers find they often need all their skills of communication to ensure a successful outcome to the scanning procedure. Patients may be allowed to play their own music tapes over the intercom which can aid in relaxation, and patients are given a panic button which they can press if they become particularly anxious during the scan itself. Scan times have reduced as equipment advances, but can still be comparatively long, and again this is an important factor. Children may need sedation to allow the scan to be performed successfully.

Summary

The complementary imaging modalities are increasingly a part of the range of diagnostic imaging investigations and many student radiographers will go on to specialize in one of these modalities. O'Connor comments that, from her clinical observations, '... such high technological methods can be depersonalizing and threatening to the patient in care who may already be anxious due to a disease process.' As part of the recommendations of her research she concludes that students should:

- 'Have an awareness of the feelings of fear, anxiety and the severe emotional distress of patients;
- Be brought to an understanding of each patient's emotional state;

- Develop observational skills allowing them to interpret accurately patients' behaviour;
- Have the ability to empathize with patients and foster a positive attitude to their illness'

(O'Connor, 1993, p 11)

References

Bryan, G. (1987) *Diagnostic Radiography – A Concise Practical Manual*, (Chapter 14), 4th Edn., Churchill Livingstone, Edinburgh.

Crawley, M. (1992) Radiologist/patient watching in ultrasound. *Research in Radiography*, 2 (1), 29–38.

Ehrlich, R.A. & McCloskey, E.D. (1989) *Patient Care in Radiography*, (pages 220–228), 3rd Edn., CV Mosby Co.

McLellan, M. (1990) The radiographer and the well-woman. *Radiography Today*, 56 (640), 26.

O'Connor, G. (1993) Social and communication skills of staff as perceived by patients during MRI. *Radiography Today*, 59 (670), 9–11.

Robinson, A. (1992) Expectation and satisfaction in patients referred for CT Scanning. *Radiography Today*, 61 (662), 13–16.

Thorp, D., Owens, R.G., Whitehouse, G. & Dewey, M.E. (1990), Subjective experiences of magnetic resonance imaging. *Clinical Radiology*, 41, 276–8.

Chapter 14
Work with Trauma and Acutely Ill Patients

Introduction

As indicated in Chapter 1, the student quickly discovers that not all patients are able to walk down to the Department and to co-operate in their examination to the extent that is encountered in the early stages of their clinical education. One of the most challenging areas of radiography (but also often the most satisfying) is the examination of acutely ill patients who may come to the Department via the accident and emergency unit suffering from trauma or other acute symptoms, or the examination of patients on the wards or intensive care units or in the operating theatres with mobile equipment. As Drafke (1990, p 1) states, 'This is no time for "learning by accident".' Radiographers in this situation need to draw on all the skills at their disposal in order to provide the highest level of patient care which these patients demand.

Work with trauma patients

As discussed earlier, trauma patients are more demanding to examine, and Fig. 14.1 reminds us of the model of the radiographic process which can help in the structuring of a trauma examination. Patient *assessment* is important and the patient's condition may require constant observation during the examination. There may be a nurse with the patient and they may have intravenous drips *in situ*, oxygen being administered and other factors which may need to be considered. *Planning* of the examination is therefore critical. Drafke (1990, p 2) states that the radiographer needs skills of planning, organization and nonverbal communication. If multiple projections are required then all the anteroposterior projections should be taken first and then the laterals. Planning of the examination helps save time and if the patient is critically injured then *speed and efficiency* in this situation are paramount. *Patient care and communication* are also very important. The patient may be anxious, confused and possibly only semi-conscious. Drafke reminds us that our own nonverbal communication is also important:

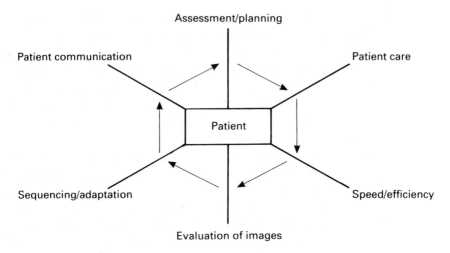

Fig. 14.1 The radiographic process.

'The radiographer must be careful not to show alarm, shock or surprise at the patient's condition. This is particularly true when the trauma has caused facial disfigurement. The radiographer must convey compassion and concern, not shock'

(Drafke, 1990, p 4)

Careful *evaluation of images* is necessary at the end of the examination. In some departments this may now include a comment on the appearances of the radiographs under the protocols of what have become known as 'Red Dot Systems'. Such systems involve radiographers placing a red adhesive spot onto any image which in their opinion has the appearance of some abnormality such as a fracture. Red dot protocols are restricted to qualified radiographers with a specified length of experience (see Appendix 1). Even where such protocols are not in operation the quality of the images is crucial and is the responsibility of the radiographer. Factors such as movement unsharpness are a major consideration in trauma; but students are reminded that radiation dose is also important and therefore films must only be repeated if by doing so the image quality and the diagnostic value **will be substantially** improved (Cullinan, 1992, Chapter 1).

Work with mobile equipment in the ward

Requests for radiography with a mobile set will reach the X-ray department from both medical and surgical wards. Medical cases are generally X-rayed in the ward because they are too ill to come to the department, and the examination most often requested is a plain film of the chest. Surgical cases will include as well as those who are too ill to come to the department a proportion of patients who are unable to leave their beds because they are secured to a frame which is applying traction to a fracture. Such patients, especially if they are young and agile and have had time to get used to the traction, often present a lively appearance and are able to co-operate with the radiographer very well within the limits of their defined area of movement.

Having arrived at the ward with the necessary equipment, the radiographer should first report to the nurse in charge and announce which patient is to be X-rayed, and the examination to be done. This is not only a courtesy to the person in charge but will enable the radiographer to find out in which part of the ward is the patient to be X-rayed, and also to receive any special information concerning the person – for example, the extent to which they may be asked to co-operate by sitting up and moving about the bed. If the patient is very ill, the nurse may feel that the radiographer should have the assistance of one of the nurses who is familiar with the patient and their treatment. It is not difficult, therefore, to see the importance of telling those in charge when the examination is being made.

It is a kindness to the patient to go in and give an explanation of what is to be undertaken. Obviously it requires a little more time and effort to do this before fetching in the equipment, but it is certainly of benefit to the patient and is not entirely without value to the radiographer. These few minutes will enable the radiographer to assess the patient's capacity for co-operation and any special difficulties which are present – for example, traction frames. Perhaps at this stage the need for assistance from the ward staff may become obvious, and it can then be sought.

Clearly it is not possible to do the radiography without *some* disturbance to the patient, and the aim should be to make this as little as is compatible with an efficient examination. Few of us fully realize what busy lives some patients lead. The doctors' rounds, visits from the physiotherapist, the performance of various special examinations and tests such as the taking of blood and other specimens for laboratory investigation – all of these may leave the patient with the impression that they are getting hardly any rest at all.

The patient should be given privacy for the X-ray examination, and either screens or cubicle curtains should be pulled round the bed. After the radiographer has finished, the patient should be made as comfortable as possible in a bed restored to neatness. The equipment should be put away with the supply cable tidily coiled and the tube column and tube head locked in a position which prevents dangerous projection before it is taken from the ward.

When accidents happen with X-ray equipment they more probably involve mobile equipment than fixed installations in departments. This is doubtless because the equipment is mobile and is taken into various situations. It becomes subject to much mechanical stress and can be the worse for lack of attention and lack of thought by its human users.

Many special conditions will be met in using a mobile set, and indeed every excursion may seem to present a challenge to technical ability. However, there are certain features with regard to the patient which are likely to recur, and an indication of these may be given here as some guidance to the student.

The patient having oxygen therapy

The need for giving the patient additional oxygen and methods of administration are discussed somewhat more fully in Chapter 9 of this book. Here it can be said that patients having continuous oxygen therapy for a period will be encountered in the wards. The oxygen is supplied from a cylinder or through a piped supply to the patient's bedside, and it is administered in one of three ways:

(1) By means of a mask fitting over the mouth and nose (see Chapter 9, Fig. 9.2);
(2) Via nasal cannulae;
(3) By means of an oxygen tent or, in the case of babies, by an oxyhood (Adler & Carlton, 1994, pp 190–191).

There are two important points to remember when doing radiography on patients who are having oxygen. Firstly, the risk of fire. The use of any electrical apparatus carries the risk of a spark when the equipment is functioning, so that it is important that while the X-ray set is operating the oxygen supply is switched off and discontinued.

The second point arises from this need to stop the supply of oxygen in order to use the X-ray set. The patient having oxygen therapy is likely to be very ill and dependent on the supply of oxygen to ameliorate his condition. It will therefore cause distress if not actual harm if the patient is without it for an appreciable time. If the radiography is to cause the patient the least disturbance, then all must be made ready with regard to the X-ray set and the patient before the oxygen supply is cut off, so that this is done for the shortest possible time.

If the patient is receiving oxygen through nasal catheters, the supply is turned off, the catheters being left in place; if by mask, the supply is cut off and the mask removed; if in a tent, the supply is cut off and the patient is taken out of the tent for the required period. It is not likely that this procedure will be left entirely to the radiographer, for it is the responsibility of the ward staff to see that the patient is receiving the oxygen correctly at the prescribed rate of flow. In the case of an oxygen tent which has been opened, it is usual for a short period afterwards to increase the rate of flow of the gas through it in order to raise the oxygen concentration.

If a member of the nursing staff is not required to give assistance with the patient throughout the X-ray examination, the radiographer's responsibility in regard to the oxygen supply may be summarized as being first to see that it is turned off before the X-ray set operates, and secondly to see that the ward staff are informed *immediately* the radiography is finished so that the oxygen supply can be restored.

The reader should turn to Chapter 9 for accounts of the risks associated with the use of oxygen and of the observations which a radiographer must make of the patient and the equipment. Here we emphasize that a radiographer working with mobile X-ray apparatus must be quick and precise in action so that the interruption in the treatment and the demands on the patient are minimal.

The patient with a drainage system

Systems for the drainage of various body cavities will be encountered during work in the wards, particularly in the surgical wards. The patient has a length of plastic or rubber tubing inserted into whichever cavity it is required to drain. In modern practice the container for any fluid which is being drained may be a plastic bag hanging from the side of the patient's bed; the bag has a metal frame at its upper edge with hooks that hang on the side of the bed. The bag may be marked with a scale to show how much fluid is in it.

A different system for the drainage of surgical wounds is a closed system of suction drainage which uses a special bottle on which a vacuum is maintained. At the end of the surgical operation which the patient has undergone, a drainage tube is inserted and left with one end inside the wound and the other protruding externally. The special vacuum bottle is then attached to the external or exit end of the drainage tube and the vacuum acts to suck out the fluid that is to be drained. The stopper of the bottle carries two little antennae which show the state of the vacuum. If there is a vacuum the two antennae are directed apart from each other like the sides of the letter V; when the vacuum is lost they come together as if the vee had been turned upside down thus Λ. This shows that the bottle needs replacing (Walsh, 1989a).

The urinary bladder may be drained by means of a catheter inserted through the urethra, and this may be done if the patient is unable to pass urine naturally, or if it is wished to keep the bladder empty and unexpanded.

The catheter may be of the self-retaining type or may be inserted supra-pubically, and the urine drains continuously away.

In approaching such patients, the principles of care should by now suggest themselves to the student from indications previously given. It is necessary to notice the presence of any external containers and to avoid striking them or compressing tubes with the X-ray equipment. In moving the patient tubing must be watched to see that it does not get kinked and that the drainage system does not become open in any way. Care must be taken to see that strain is not put on the tubing. This increases the risk of the tube coming out and of connections pulling apart, and in some cases may cause the patient pain.

The patient on traction

The word traction means the act of drawing or pulling and patients encountered in hospital may be 'on traction' as part of their treatment. This involves applying a pulling force to some structure: for instance, in the treatment of fractures overriding broken bones may be pulled apart in the correction of displacements; muscle spasm may be relieved by a pulling force applied to a limb. The pulling force is achieved by the use of weights suspended above the ground in weight carriers so that the applied force is that of gravity (Heywood-Jones, 1990). There are:

(1) Skin traction;
(2) Skeletal traction.

Skin traction may be used to relieve muscle spasm or temporarily to immobilize a limb. The force is applied to the skin, for example, by fixing elastoplast to the inner and outer sides of a leg from just above the ankle to mid-thigh and bandaging with an elasticated bandage. Weights can be applied to the elastoplast traction, the weights being suspended in a carrier by means of a cord passing over a pulley as shown in Fig. 14.2. The pull of the weights towards the ground is transmitted to the elastoplast traction and hence to the affected limb.

In **skeletal traction** the pulling force is applied directly to a long bone. A metal pin is driven through the bone: this is a surgical procedure undertaken in the operating theatre with the patient given a general anaesthetic. A curved piece of metal called a stirrup is fixed securely to the protruding ends of the pin, the exposed points of the pin being finally covered by guards. The traction is again achieved by suspended weights and is applied through the stirrup and pin as shown in Fig. 14.3.

Patients on traction frequently have the end of bed raised on blocks in order to put a slope on it. There may be an overhead beam with pulleys.

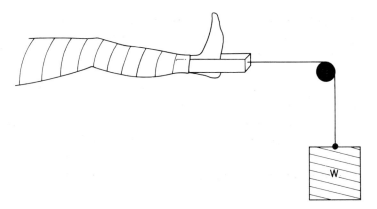

Fig. 14.2 Skin traction.

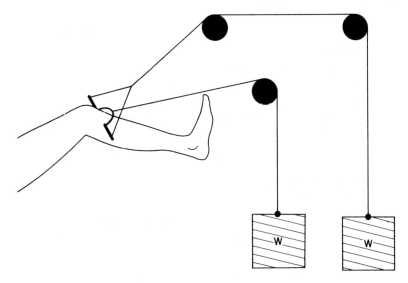

Fig. 14.3 Skeletal traction.

Approaching such a patient, the radiographer should observe the presence both of the blocks underneath the bed and of any overhead framework. Failure to appreciate these features may result in the bed being pulled off the blocks by an unobservant attempt to move it, and in the X-ray tube head being crashed against the overhead structures as the mobile set is wheeled into position.

Since any weights applied are intended to give a continuous pull, they must not be lifted or allowed to rest on anything so that the cord holding them becomes slack.

Limbs being supported in splints for the application of traction will be seen to rest in broad flannel slings, arranged so that each sling has its proximal edge overlapped by the distal edge of the one above it; this prevents any pressure from the edges. The slings are attached to the splint by 'bulldog' clips. These are likely to obscure certain radiographic projections, and they may with due care be replaced by safety pins for the period of the X-ray examination.

Giving a patient a bedpan

The use of a bedpan is probably one of the procedures most dreaded and disliked by any patient who contemplates a period in hospital in the course of which they may be immobilized in bed. This is a very understandable view.

In the first place, a male patient will be embarrassed about asking for the bedpan when he needs it. According to his age, he may feel that a young nurse (junior nurses who deal with bedpans tend to be young!) is too nearly the age of his grandchildren, or of his children, or of his own friends for him easily to be able to mention such basic functions to her. A woman patient may escape the embarrassment but may share a reluctance to make a demand on busy nurses and a worry as to whether the nurse will bring the bedpan in time to prevent the delay making itself disastrously evident in the bed.

In the second place, once the patient is on the bedpan he finds it difficult to use, and this of course applies to women patients too. A patient supine in bed, or a patient sitting up in bed on a bedpan which is balanced on a yielding mattress, is in a position very different from those assumed naturally for the performance of the functions with which the use of the bedpan is associated. It is difficult to use the abdominal muscles effectively. There may be a feeling of insecurity and a fear of falling which tend to impair concentration on the physical functions. So for various reasons the bedpan is a disliked object.

In modern hospital practice the bedpan is used only when it *must* be. Patients who can walk to the lavatory are encouraged to do so, and certainly need little encouragement in most cases. Those who are able just to get out of bed can use commode chairs which are brought to the bedside. A commode chair is a chair which can take a bedpan in the place of its seat and a patient using it finds it much more like using an ordinary lavatory. Even those on complete bed-rest are often today allowed to get out of bed and use a commode chair because the effort and worry of this are much less than those associated with the use of the bedpan in bed. However, it is clear that bedpans must be used sometimes, and it is useful if radiographers in the X-ray department know how to deal with them.

The first step is to ensure privacy for the patient; a sense of lack of privacy is one of the trials of life to a patient in the hospital ward. The patient should use the bedpan in a room which affords privacy and not, for example, in a waiting bay or corridor surrounded by other patients. The bedpan should be brought to the patient with a cover over it. In modern hospital practice this cover is disposable, being paper, and its once-only use is a great aid to hygiene.

The bedpan should be clean and dry and neither too hot nor too cold. A cold pan is uncomfortable but is not so dangerous as a pan which is too hot. Carrying a bedpan, the radiographer should hold it firmly with both hands, keeping it away from all contact with the unprotected uniform coat; this is important for reasons of hygiene. Unlike nurses, radiographers do not usually have to issue a number of bedpans at a time and are therefore spared the temptation to load themselves up with a pile which is desperately clutched to their chests and abdomens in order to prevent the pans falling.

Two radiographers assist patients who cannot help themselves. They place themselves one on each side of the patient; the radiographer at the patient's left side puts her right arm under the patient's body at just below waist level, and the one on the patient's right side puts her left arm in a similar position. One radiographer then puts a free hand under the upper part of the patient's thighs and together they raise the patient's body. This may be facilitated with the aid of lifting slings or similar (see Chapter 2). The radiographer with one hand still free uses it to push the bedpan from the side to a position under the patient's buttocks. Figure 14.4 indicates the placing of the bedpan for a supine patient; if the 'front end' is not visible at the patient's crotch the bedpan is too far up the body to be useful.

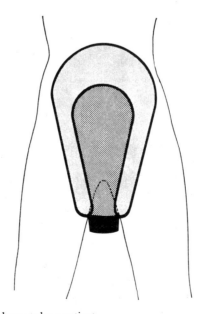

Fig. 14.4 Placing a bedpan under a patient.

It may take two radiographers and four hands to lift a patient who is very heavy, while a third radiographer puts the bedpan in place. If the patient is able to rise to a sitting position, it is of course easy for one radiographer to manage the procedure unaided. Should the patient be able to sit up on the bedpan, care should be given to preventing the possibility of a fall, particularly if the person is liable to feel faint or dizzy or is not agile. Toilet paper should be available to be used.

When the bedpan has been used it should be removed by manoeuvres similar to those which placed it. The patient should be made comfortable and should be given the means – a bowl of warm water, soap and a paper towel – with which to wash and dry their hands.

The patient may have used the bedpan simply to evacuate an enema received in the X-ray department as preparation for or as part of a diagnostic procedure. In this case, once the results have been noted the bedpan, unless it is disposable, may be emptied down the lavatory and then washed and sterilized in readiness for further use. Disposable bedpans and urinals require special machinery for their disposal. The patient may be on a regime which involves saving excreta through 24 hours for various tests or measuring urinary output. The radiographer should ascertain from the ward what must be done in regard to urine and faeces that may be passed while the patient is in the X-ray department.

Work with mobile equipment in the operating theatre

When a radiographer undertakes an examination using mobile equipment in an operating theatre, this work is regarded as being of an emergency nature, and the time factor is important. The aim always in surgical procedures is to be as quick as is consistent with efficiency, for prolonging the length of time that the patient is undergoing surgery and is kept under anaesthesia increases the risk. The burden of responsibility for the patient's well-being which rests upon the surgeon makes him exacting in his requirements and the radiographer must be prepared to produce good radiographs without delay.

There are many technical features to be considered, but they are not within the scope of this book, and discussion will be limited to some general principles relative to operating theatre technique and the patient's safety.

On first going to the theatre, the radiographer must check that all the required equipment has been brought and is ready for use, and that the X-ray set is plugged into the right power supply and is working correctly.

Explosion risk in the operating theatre

Although it may be something which does not impress itself immediately on the newcomer to the operating theatre, there is an explosion risk present due to the use for anaesthesia of gases which readily ignite or promote ignition. It has therefore been considered important to reduce the chance of a spark occurring, and in designing equipment for the theatre attention has been paid to this point.

Possible sources of ignition which suggest themselves are hot surfaces such as theatre spotlights and bulbs, and all electrical instruments which may be used in the theatre. A less noticeable but equally important source is due to the phenomenon known as static electricity.

Static electricity is present all the time. It is produced when insulated objects have friction applied to them, even if this friction is only that given by passing through the air. Very high potentials or electrical 'pressures' can be produced, and when two objects which have acquired electric charge in this way are brought close to each other, charge is transferred from one to the other. The object which is at the higher potential will transfer electric charge to the one at lower potential, and this creates a spark. The spark may be very small and not perceived by the eye, but even an infinitely small spark can cause an explosion in an atmosphere filled with flammable gases.

Various safety 'anti-static' devices and precautions are used, the aim being to keep everything in the theatre if possible at the same electrical potential or pressure, and to try to prevent the accumulation of static electricity. Many operating theatres are now designed with floors which will conduct electricity and allow it to leak slowly away. Stretcher trolleys have sometimes been given a length of chain which drags on the floor as they are pushed about the hospital, and provides a pathway for the dispersal of the electric charge which they might otherwise collect; some of them have 'anti-static' wheels. Certain synthetic fibres show readiness to acquire electric charge. In some theatres the wearing of nylon underclothing is forbidden to the theatre staff on duty.

X-ray equipment operates at high voltages, and no matter what safety precautions exist in the theatre itself no one can guarantee that the X-ray apparatus is spark-proof. It is part of the radiographer's responsibility to understand, and to see that others understand, the risk involved in using X-ray equipment in conjunction with gases which readily ignite or promote ignition. Surgical procedures which require radiography should be taken with anaesthetic gases not flammable in character.

Surgical asepsis in the operating theatre

Explanation has already been given of the risks of infection to patients during surgery (Chapter 4), and of the need to undertake surgical procedures in conditions of asepsis which exclude the presence of living organisms. When mobile X-ray equipment is brought to the operating theatre there is not only added risk of explosion, but threat to the sterility of conditions of the operating field.

The mobile equipment should be reserved exclusively for use in the theatre but unfortunately it may instead move throughout the hospital, collecting fluff and dust from the wards as it goes. It is thus a potential carrier of bacteria, and it is furthermore a piece of equipment which it is impossible to sterilize completely.

It is preferable if some mobile equipment can be kept permanently within the theatre suite. The advantages of this practice are:

(1) That the equipment is immediately available for use;
(2) The risks of bringing infection to the theatre are reduced.

It is the radiographer's responsibility to see the X-ray set and accessories are clean and free from dust. Since the X-ray tube head in many instances will be placed directly over the operating field, particular attention should be paid to it. In some theatres it may be the practice to enclose the tube head and any image intensifier in a sterile linen or polythene cover, and this is one way of making quite sure that no particles fall into the field of operation.

With regard to personal clothing in the operating theatre, the radiographer must follow the rules applying to theatre staff. Almost certainly a clean gown, a face mask and covering for the head will be issued, together with some form of special footwear (such as pumps, rubber boots, or cotton coverings to tie over the shoes). All these are designed to ensure that the radiographer does not bring into the theatre bacteria from other parts of the hospital.

The theatre may be considered as having two areas:

(1) The sterile area,
(2) The non-sterile area.

The *sterile area* is primarily the operation field, and in it are included the patient and the operation wound, the surgeon and his immediate assistants (both medical and nursing staff), all the instruments and equipment which they will directly handle, and any trays, trolleys, or tables which hold equipment in readiness for them.

The rest of the theatre constitutes the *non-sterile area*. In it are the anaesthetist and his equipment from which the anaesthetic gases are supplied, the rest of the theatre staff, and diverse accessory equipment. The radiographer and the X-ray machine work in this non-sterile area.

Those working in the theatre have a duty to see that no contamination of the *sterile* area occurs from the *non-sterile area*. The radiographer must be careful not to touch, either personally or with any of the X-ray apparatus and accessories, anything in the theatre which is sterile. This will need care in the manipulation of the mobile set and in positioning cassettes. Movement about the theatre should be restricted to avoid disturbance of the air; this might carry organisms from the floor and other non-sterile regions into a sterile field. Similarly to reduce the risk of droplet contamination, talk in the operating theatre should be kept within the limits of necessity.

Traditionally, when the surgeon views radiographs he moves from the sterile area in the immediate vicinity of the operating table out to the non-sterile area in order to get close to the X-ray illuminator. It will be seen that he is careful not to contaminate himself by touching his gown or his hands against anything not sterile; he will hold his hands folded together in front of him. The radiographer must be equally careful not to contaminate the surgeon as the radiographs are being shown. Increasingly theatre radiography is undertaken as a fluoroscopic examination using a mobile image intensifier and coupled television system, which allows the surgeon to view images without the need to move out of the sterile area. Radiation dose can also be reduced by the use of pulsed fluoroscopy, and image retention (memory) devices can help significantly in dose reduction to the patient (Carter, 1994).

The sterile areas in the theatre are often distinguished by special coloration, all the towels, gowns, and drapes over the patient or trolleys being coloured green (in some cases blue) so that there is visual reminder of their sterility.

Radiation safety

Radiation risk to the patient during radiographic examinations is discussed more fully in another part of this book (Chapter 19). It cannot be too strongly emphasized that wherever X-ray equipment is being used by a radiographer the responsibility for radiation safety rests on that radiographer, unless a radiologist is present and is taking charge of the examination. The radiographer *must* see that the conditions of use are safe and that the patient and staff are not excessively or unnecessarily exposed to X-rays; this may entail giving an authoritative opinion to senior people highly trained in their own specialty but not trained in the use of X-rays.

The Ionizing Radiations Regulations (1985 & 1988) state that when a mobile unit is connected to the mains supply a controlled area shall exist around the unit to a distance of 2 metres and that the use of the unit must be covered by a written system of work. The radiographer operating the unit must have a clear view of the controlled area and must given an audible warning that an exposure is about to take place.

No one other than the patient under examination must be in the line of the direct beam. This point requires particular attention when the beam is directed horizontally and may include in its range patients in adjoining beds and staff in the ward or operating theatre. If necessary, beds must be moved away and staff should be warned to keep clear while the exposure is made.

The radiographer should wear a lead-rubber apron. Any supporting of the patient should be done by a nurse or other non-radiographic staff (not the same assistant too often), and a lead-rubber apron and if necessary gloves should be worn and the details recorded in a book located on the mobile machine. This is a precaution to ensure that the same members of staff are not being repeatedly irradiated.

With recognition of the sources of risk and careful attention to these relatively simple precautions, the use of mobile equipment should have a level of protection equivalent to that available to the radiographer at work in the X-ray department.

Major accident procedure

It is unfortunately the case that there are occasions when the Accident & Emergency and Imaging departments need to make special provision for an influx of trauma patients. Walsh (1989b) defines a disaster as:

'... a situation in which normal resources can no longer cope. A disaster plan therefore allows the mobilization of sufficient extra resources, as quickly as possible'.

In the case of incidents such as fires or crashes, the designation of a major accident (incident) is made by the first senior officer of the emergency services on the scene. In many cases the determination that the disaster should be designated in this way depends upon the number of live casualties. Individual disaster plans are developed for each town, city or geographical area and are tailored to the circumstances of the particular locality. For example, cities such as Manchester must take account of Manchester Airport, the heavily concentrated motorway network which surrounds the city and industrial considerations such as chemical works, where there may be the possibility of an explosion. Disaster planning is done as a collaborative enterprise between the various emergency services and certain hospitals within a geographical area will be designated for the reception of casualties. Various hospitals may be involved with, for example, neurosurgical centres being designated for the receipt of head injury patients and other patients with different injuries being taken to general hospitals. The efficient working of such a plan relies on *TRIAGE* of casualties at the accident site. That is, the sorting of patients by the type and extent of their injury to determine priorities for treatment (Tattum, 1987).

In any hospital designated to be involved in a major incident, it is the responsibility of the imaging services manager to devise an individual plan for the involvement of the imaging department. Students are advised to look at the plans for their own placement departments. The plan will vary depending upon whether the disaster occurs during working hours or at night (when there may only be one on-call radiographer initially available). The imaging services manager must be informed as soon as possible of the type and extent of the incident and of the expected number of casualties and their potential time of arrival (Fawcett, 1987). If the incident takes place at night then a cascade system is instituted whereby staff initially informed are instructed to ring other members of the department and to call them in as required. This may be on a staged basis so that staff can be relieved by personnel who are rested. During the day, non-urgent cases are likely to be re-booked and the department is cleared as required to allow for the reception and efficient throughput of the expected casualties. As Walsh (1989b) states, 'The plan must establish a clear chain of command. A disaster is no place for arguing about who does what'. The Major Incident plans are reviewed at regular intervals and practices may also be instituted to check that the plan will operate effectively. This is important as, thankfully, such incidents are still comparatively rare.

References

Adler, A.M. & Carlton, R. (1994) *Introduction to Radiography and Patient Care*, (pages 190–191), WB Saunders Co, Philadelphia.

Carter, P. (1994) *Chesney's Equipment for Student Radiographers*, (Chapter 7), 4th Edn., Blackwell Science, Oxford.

Cullinan, A.M. (1992) *Optimizing Radiographic Positioning*, (Chapter 1), JB Lippincott Co, Philadelphia.

Drafke, M. (1990) *Trauma and Mobile Radiography*, (pages 1–4), FA Davis Co.

Fawcett, J. (1987) Diary of a disaster. *Nursing Times*, 83 (43), 28–30.

Heywood Jones, I. (1990) Making sense of traction. *Nursing Times*, 86 (23), 39–41.

Tattum, A. (1987) Lessons from King's Cross. *Nursing Standard*, Dec 12th, 28.

Walsh, M. (1989a) Making sense of chest drainage. *Nursing Times*, 85 (24), 40–41.

Walsh, M. (1989b) Coping with catastrophe. *Nursing Times*, 85 (19), 27–31.

Chapter 15
The Infectious Patient

The student will by now appreciate the risks of cross infection in hospital and understand procedures designed to prevent any patient from acquiring an infection in hospital. As well as the detailed techniques of surgical asepsis (which can form only a small part of the radiographer's daily duties), attention must be paid to general considerations of hygiene in the X-ray department; these are not less important than techniques for asepsis. Many patients for X-ray examination will not be involved during the course of it in surgical procedures; *all* patients will be dependent on departmental practice in hygiene to protect them against infection.

Hygiene in the X-ray department

Although considerations of hygiene may be rated as secondary in a state of emergency, nevertheless the general practice of hygiene in the X-ray department is an important factor in care of the patient.

In this case the risk against which the patient is to be protected is cross infection – that is the acquiring of an infection which he did not have when he came to the hospital. It is important to protect from infection not only the patient but also the staff, and conditions of hygiene directed for the patient's benefit will assist also the staff. However, the staff have on their side the advantage of a tendency to acquire *immunity*, whereas the tendency of the patient is to acquire *infection*. He/she is already in a state of lowered resistance and is susceptible to invasion by bacteria.

The successful prevention of cross infection in hospitals depends upon every single member of its staff, not only those who handle patients but those who handle materials which will be in contact with patients and ward and departmental clinical staff. Much attention to detail is required from all concerned. For example, a laundry-bag can bring infection to the ward because at some stage in its transport it has been allowed to rest on the ground in the hospital yard.

As a contribution to general departmental hygiene, radiographers should pay attention to personal hygiene. Short clean nails, clean and tidy hair, clean shoes, and a fresh white coat are less likely to carry and transmit disease. Hands washed between the handling of patients, and after contact with such articles as bedpans, urinals, used instruments, dressings, etc., should be a practised routine so customary that it does not need to be remembered (Gidley, 1987).

Hygiene for the patient must be maintained by ensuring that he/she has a clean gown to wear and a clean cubicle in which to undress. In the X-ray room clean linen and blankets should be provided for the X-ray table. Disposable paper sheets of various sizes are useful here, since they can be laid over the pillow case and over a linen sheet where the patient lies and fresh ones supplied for each patient.

Any utensils given to the patient – for example bedpans, urinals, receivers, drinking mugs, containers for dentures, etc. – must be clean. In modern practice many of these items are disposable. These are a great aid to hygiene as they are used only once (although there is a resource implication in not attempting to re-sterilize such items).

The radiolucent plastic foam pads which are accessories frequently found in X-ray departments should be washed often, and may conveniently be enclosed in polythene sheeting to save them from contamination by blood and other discharges. For drying the hands, ordinary roller towels should not be used as they provide a medium favourable to bacterial growth, and they should be replaced by disposable paper towels, or the type of towel dispenser which continuously provides a fresh area of towel for each user.

The X-ray rooms and changing rooms should be well ventilated and must be kept clean and tidy. Accessories such as the pads previously mentioned should be kept in closed cupboards where they are more likely to escape dust. The top of the X-ray table and the front surface of the erect bucky stand should be cleaned down with a suitable antiseptic solution and particular attention should be paid to this if the patient has been in direct contact with it, as may occur in radiography of the skull and sinuses.

Aerosol sprays are very useful here as they allow quick, easy and hygienic application of the cleansing agent. It is good practice to keep an aerosol container of antiseptic in the X-ray room where skull and sinus examinations are carried out, together with a supply of disposable tissues for wiping dry the sprayed area. All such cleaning must be carried out wearing disposable gloves, to avoid contact with body fluids which may have been deposited on the table top.

It is part of the radiographer's responsibility to see that the department is clean, even if it is not necessary for the radiographer actually to undertake much cleaning. In most cases general cleaning will be done by the hospital cleaners, but the work of cleaning equipment and various accessories will be taken by the radiographer. No one should find the task beneath professional dignity, for the maintenance of clean conditions is an important part of departmental care, and is related to our responsibility towards the patient.

Routines of cleanliness both for staff and patients must be unremittingly undertaken. Disregard of detail in this leads to generally careless practice which increases everyone's risk – particularly that of the patient, who is more susceptible and more exposed. It may be assumed here that this general care is applied to all patients. Patients known to have a disease communicable to others require particular additional precautions.

The spread of infection

Communicable diseases may be spread in various ways. If the question is asked: 'What is infectious about a patient?' the following have to be considered in the answer.

(1) Droplet discharge from patient's nose and mouth;
(2) Faeces;
(3) Urine and other body fluids, especially where they contain visible blood;
(4) Sputum;
(5) Discharge from wounds, sores, and body cavities.

As examples, the organisms of anterior poliomyelitis and cerebrospinal meningitis are contained in the nose and throat secretions of those who have the diseases, and may be conveyed by droplets when such a patient coughs, breathes, and talks. In other diseases, such as typhoid fever and dysentery, the infectious materials are the patient's excreta (urine and faeces) from which infection may be conveyed to bedpans, bed linen, and other things. The bacteria of pulmonary tuberculosis are contained in the sputum. Some bacteria can live in the dried state.

Communicable diseases can be spread by direct contact between the patient and other people; also through an intermediary, an article which has been in contact with the patient. All things in contact with the patient can be considered as infected because of contamination which may reach them directly, may be airborne, may be conveyed by the patient's hands, and may reach them from other articles previously infected. This process is illustrated in Fig. 15.1.

In caring for such patients, isolation technique is designed to stop the spread of the disease to other people by close control of the area within which contact occurs. The word contact in this sense embraces all three elements – the patient, other people, and things.

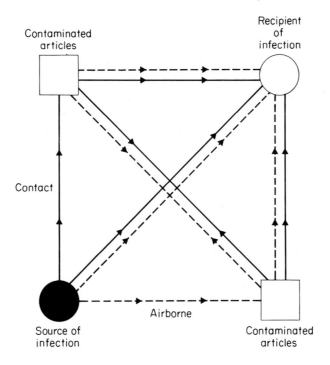

Fig. 15.1 Illustration of the spread of infection. *(Copy from Staphylococcal Infection in Hospitals, by kind permission of the controller of HM Stationery Office.)*

The infectious patient in the X-ray department

The increasing prevalence of HIV and AIDS in the late 1980s caused employers to review their practices for handling patients. Both HIV and hepatitis B (which in fact presents a far greater risk to the health care worker than HIV or AIDS) can be transmitted by symptomless carriers. In accordance with the Health & Safety at Work Act, therefore, each trust board has a legal responsibility to institute what have become known as 'universal precautions' for the handling of blood and body fluids. These precautions are embodied for the radiography profession in the Control of Infection Protocol, published by the College of Radiographers (1990). The protocol underlines the fact that:

'Since it is not always known whether a patient may be carrying either hepatitis B virus (HBV) or human immunodeficiency virus (HIV) ALL blood and body fluids from ALL patients must be treated as potentially hazardous' (College of Radiographers, 1990).

The College protocol suggests the following mandatory routine to be followed with all patients who are known to be suffering from a dangerous infection **and** for all patients who are

'... bleeding or likely to bleed, incontinent, vomiting, suffering from open skin lesions, unconscious or mentally disturbed or confused'.

(College of Radiographers, 1990)

If possible the infectious patient should not be allowed to come to the X-ray department, but should be examined by means of a mobile X-ray set taken to the ward. If an infectious patient does come to the X-ray department, they must be there for the shortest time consistent with an efficient examination, and they must be kept away from other patients while in the department. If there is choice of time, then this should be at a period when the department is not busy and there are few other patients present. This will make it easier to ensure the isolation of the infectious one, and the lack of pressure from other work will expedite the processing of films and their subsequent viewing. Thus the patient will not be kept long in the department. If there is little or no choice of the time, then the patient must be given priority over other patients, and must be X-rayed on arrival in the department. After the examination it will probably be necessary to ask the patient to wait a little time until the films are viewed, and they should be isolated from other patients during this period, which should be made as brief as possible.

When the patient comes to the X-ray room, it should be ready with the table covered with a fresh disposable sheet and the pillow similarly protected.

If the patient is to be put in direct contact with the cassette, or positioned against a vertical bucky stand or cassette holder, disposable coverings should be available for these. Any linen or disposable coverings used for this patient should be removed as soon as the examination is finished.

The number of people involved in the examination should be minimized and staff should wear gowns, plastic aprons and plastic gloves. If there is any likelihood of splashing of blood then additional protection in the form of mask and plastic goggles is also advised.

Spillage of blood or other body fluids on the table top or other surface should be covered immediately with an appropriate disinfectant. The College of Radiographers' protocol recommends two examples of appropriate disinfectants but in particular hospitals these are likely to be specified by the Trust Board in their own code of practice. Whichever disinfectant is used, it should be left to act for 5 minutes before being cleared up with gloves worn and using disposable wipes.

If the patient has to wait for films to be viewed before the examination is declared complete, it is really better that they should wait in the X-ray room, even although this may delay the use of the room for other patients. Once the X-ray room has been given over to the examination of the infectious patient, it is more truly careful of the others to keep them waiting a little longer until this examination is complete and the patient has left the department.

A radiographer working unaided is clearly required to handle accessories and the controls of the X-ray set as well as the patient; this necessitates a careful disinfecting afterwards of *everything* with which the radiographer or the patient has been in contact. This must include cassettes manipulated by the radiographer, the controls of the X-ray set, the tube head and tube column. The cassettes must be thoroughly and carefully wiped with disinfectant before being taken into the processing room. A hygienic way of using the antiseptic or disinfectant is to apply it as an aerosol spray and wipe with a disposable tissue. The radiographer in a contaminated state should try to handle cassettes as little as possible, touching them only by the corners and edges.

It will be better if the radiographer can work with an assistant. The radiographer will help and position the patient, and the assistant will manipulate the equipment, set the controls, and make the exposure. This assistant must *not* touch the patient or anything with which the patient is in contact.

During the course of examination, it may be necessary for the radiographer who has been in contact with the patient to leave the X-ray room in order to view films. If this is so, the radiographer must remove the gown, taking care not to allow its outer aspect to make contact with the inner aspect; the outer aspect is contaminated, the inner one is 'clean'. The hands must then be well washed and scrubbed with soap and warm water before the radiographer leaves the room. It should be noticed that if the taps cannot be turned off with an elbow and there is no assistant available, the radiographer must put a tissue or disposable towel over the taps before turning them on. The towel is then discarded; once the hands are washed they may be used for manipulation of the taps, as they are now clean. On returning to the X-ray room and the patient, the radiographer must again put on the gown, observing the same precautions as when it was taken off.

When the examination is complete and the patient has left the X-ray room, the radiographer disposes of any coverings which have been in contact with the patient. If they are to be laundered, all soiled linen should be double bagged in the sacks provided by the hospital for this purpose. Clinical waste must also be double bagged in the plastic sacks designated by the hospital for the disposal of hazardous clinical waste. Usually these are coloured (yellow or red-check, whichever is in use in your own institution) to distinguish them from those used for ordinary waste. The bags should be sealed with tape, not stapled (College of Radiographers, 1990).

The radiographer then washes the hands well, removes the gown, folding it so that the inner side is outwards, washes the hands again, and removes the face mask, taking care to handle only the tapes. Mask and gown are then discarded. Attention should be given to any part of the X-ray equipment which has been contaminated by contact with the patient and the radiographer. All such parts should be cleaned thoroughly with a suitable disinfectant. Finally the hands should be well washed once again before attending to the next patient.

Handling of sharps

It is important to take particular care in the handling of sharps. Wherever possible the usage and handling of sharps should be avoided and **under no circumstances** must needles be resheathed. Sharps must be disposed of by placing them carefully into an approved sharps container which is made of rigid plastic and is usually yellow in colour and marked with a hazard warning. Such containers must be sealed and replaced when they are three-quarters full. If a needlestick or other sharps injury takes place the wound should be encouraged to bleed and the area should be thoroughly washed with warm water and soap (but **not** scrubbed). A waterproof plaster should be applied. An accident form must be completed and the occupational health department or control of infection officer must be informed. If there are splashes of body fluids into eyes, mouth or nose these should be well irrigated and again the incident must be formally reported.

Such incidents will be followed up by the taking of blood samples both from the worker involved and (if possible) from the patient themselves (College of Radiographers, 1990).

The infectious patient in the ward

Source isolation (barrier nursing)

As has been explained, it is preferable that the patient with a communicable disease should be X-rayed in the ward by means of a mobile X-ray set.

Such a patient will be nursed with an isolation technique which is called source isolation or barrier nursing. The aim of source isolation is to stop staff acquiring from a patient the infective organisms of a specific communicable disease. The patient is in a room by themselves. Usually there will be a notice on the door drawing attention to the isolation nursing; a radiographer who is in any doubt about the situation must ask the ward staff. Very occasionally the patient may be in a corner of a general ward.

Nursing staff prepare a room specially for nursing an infected patient and they consider what must be inside and what must be available immediately outside the room. The following lists indicate arrangements which are usually encountered.

Inside the room are:

(1) All the equipment required for washing;
(2) A supply of soap and paper towels at the washbasin; a small store of whatever bags (linen, plastic, paper) may be used for the disposal of contaminated items of various sorts;
(3) A commode, paper covers, disposable bedpans and urinals;
(4) A plastic bag, which is likely to be colour-coded, supported on a skip for the reception of contaminated linen.

Outside the room are:

(1) A notice which reads NO ADMISSION. ALL VISITORS TO CONSULT NURSE IN CHARGE;
(2) A table to hold the patient's charts and a supply of face-masks;
(3) A pedal bin for discarded masks;
(4) Plastic aprons, gowns and gloves;
(5) In a container, a colour-coded plastic bag for contaminated articles which are to be incinerated.

Food and drink are served on disposable plates and in plastic cups and disposable cutlery is used.

Equipment for clinical examination – such as a stethoscope and a sphygmomanometer – is kept in the room and so is a supply of linen. Everything in the patient's room is considered to be infected. Anyone who enters the patient's room and touches anything within it – including any furniture and the floor – is regarded as being in contact with infection.

Gowns and masks are provided for those who attend the patient, and the practice is for these things to be put on when entering the room and removed when leaving it. As the purpose of the gown is to prevent contamination of the clothes of the staff by which infection could be carried to other patients, it is clear that the outer and inner aspects of the gowns must not make contact with each other, as the inner is the 'clean' side. Often the outer side is clearly marked – for example by a broad band of bright colour round the hem.

In the room close to the entrance to the patient's room there will be facilities for washing the hands. The door of the patient's room should be closed after entry.

If the radiographer has to work quite unaided, then it must be recognized again that the apparatus used will become contaminated. This includes the cassette, which the radiographer must handle after it has been in contact with the patient, the controls of the mobile set, the tube column and tube head, and the supply cable which is drawn over the floor.

As in the case of an infectious patient being examined in the X-ray department, it will be better if the radiographer works with an assistant, for in this way much of the equipment can be spared contamination. This assistant should be *very* careful to avoid any physical contact with the patient, the bed, any of the furniture in the room, and those parts of the X-ray set which have been contaminated by contact with the bed and the floor. The radiographer positions the patient, and the assistant positions the X-ray tube head, sets the controls, and makes the exposure.

The cassette should be enclosed in a clean pillowcase, dressing towel, or paper towel of adequate size. After use the assistant will remove it, the radiographer holding the cassette in its wrapping in such a way that the assistant can remove the cassette without touching the outer parts of whatever has enclosed it. The assistant can then take the cassette to the processor.

If more than one cassette is to be used for the examination, the assistant must bring them in one at a time from outside the patient's room. If the radiographer is working without assistance, all the necessary cassettes must be brought into the room at the start so that the gowned radiographer does not have to pass in and out of the room several times. They will have to be safeguarded from radiation fog and must all be considered as contaminated, being thoroughly wiped with disinfectant before being taken to the processor (The disinfecting process must not be carried out with an enthusiasm that leaves the cassettes wrecked by fluid! The use of an aerosol spray with care and of disposable tissues for wiping is recommended.)

When the examination is finished and the patient is made comfortable again, the radiographer should wash the hands and then move the X-ray set away from the bed and disconnect it from the mains. The X-ray set and all contaminated parts are thoroughly cleaned with disinfectant; this includes the supply cable, which must be coiled up in its place in readiness to take the set from the room when the radiographer leaves. After leaving the room, the radiographer closes the door, discards the mask, gown and gloves, and again washes the hands.

Protective isolation (reverse barrier nursing)

Source isolation, discussed above, is a situation in which the patient is to be protected from organisms which may be carried by the staff and by visitors. The system of protection for the patient used in such a case is called reverse barrier nursing or protective isolation. Its practicalities are in fact similar to those of source isolation because they are to bar the conveyance of organisms. The difference between the two situations is the direction of travel of the organisms which it is wished to stop. In source isolation the preventable direction of travel is from the patient outwards; in the reverse technique it is to the patient inwards.

Protective isolation is required when a patient is especially susceptible to infection: so susceptible that some quite trivial infection (the common cold, for example) could prove dangerous. This can be the case when the body's resistance to infection has been lowered to an extreme degree.

Lowered resistance to infection follows whenever there is suppression of the body's normal response (the immune reaction or the immune response) to invasion by organisms or to the introduction of substances which the cells of the body want to reject. In certain cases this suppression of the immune reaction is sought deliberately. This is so, for example, in some transplant surgery where one of the problems to be met is that cells of the patient's body reject the transplanted organ because it is foreign material. In order to reduce the likelihood of such rejection, the patient's immune reaction is previously suppressed by drugs or sometimes by radiotherapy. This lack of the normal immune reaction leaves the patient most susceptible to infection.

In other cases the lowered resistance to infection accompanies some forms of treatment as an unwanted side effect. For example, the treatment of leukaemia whether by drugs or by radiotherapy reduces the number of white cells in the circulating blood. One of the functions of certain white blood cells is to ingest micro-organisms of other cells and substances as part of the body's resistance to disease or to invasion by foreign cells. With a lowered white cell count the patient becomes very susceptible to infection.

Modern treatment for various forms of malignant disease includes the use of cytotoxic drugs. The term *cytotoxic* means that these drugs can kill certain cells and the objective in using them is to kill the malignant cells (which may be very widespread) in the patient's body. An effect of their use is the killing of certain other cells as well. While being treated with these drugs the patient has a lowered white cell count in the blood and reduced ability to resist infection.

These situations call for protective isolation. For this the patient may be placed in a special room in which the air pressure is slightly positive. As a result there is no tendency for air currents to be drawn into the room, bringing with them airborne bacteria and other micro-organisms. Thus danger to the patient is effectively reduced. This positive air pressure is also used in some operating theatres.

The outlines of practical procedures in protective isolation are given below.

(1) A single room is required for the patient.
(2) Gowns, gloves and masks are worn by attending staff.
(3) Staff wash their hands before entering and then on leaving the room.

(4) Disposable crockery and cutlery are used.
(5) The patient's charts should remain outside the room.
(6) If the patient has not acquired an infection, no special precautions are necessary for the disposal of secretions and excretions.
(7) If the patient has not acquired an infection, no special precautions are necessary for the disposal of bed linen.

References

College of Radiographers (1990) *Control of Infection Protocol.*
Gidley, C. (1987) Now, wash your hands! *Nursing Times*, 83 (29), 40–42.

Further reading

Adams, M.P. (1990) Attitudes of selected radiographers towards AIDS. *Radiologic Technology*, 62 (2), 122–9.
Aitken, V. (1994) Radiographers and AIDS – do we know ourselves? *Research In Radiography*, 3 (1), 12–20.

Chapter 16
Clinical Signs and Tests

When patients come to hospital they are seeking advice on abnormalities with which they feel they need help. These deviations from the normal may be detectable in the structure or in the function of any bodily organ or system or of course may be some aberration of the mind. Radiographers are concerned rather with examinations directed to bodily abnormalities than with investigations into the infinities of the mind. In this chapter we are to interest ourselves only in patients whose problems are seated in the structures or function of their bodily organs.

Symptoms, signs and observations

What brings the patient to the doctor as a first step? Obviously, the patient seeks advice on some abnormality which they have detected themselves. 'I keep getting these awful headaches.' 'I've got this tiresome rash.' 'I've found this alarming lump.' These abnormalities that are obvious to the patient are called symptoms. As Evans (1989) states, 'Each test is a confrontation with the unknown.'

In giving this patient help, the doctor's first objective is to establish a diagnosis: that is, to identify the disease process which may be present. If treatment is to be rational and the likely future for the patient to be assessed, diagnosis is essential. Each diagnosis has its own prognosis: the term prognosis means the predictions which can be made on the course of the disease, its treatment, its termination and the recovery (or lack of recovery) which can be foreseen for the patient.

The doctors gains information by listening to what the patient has to say. This information can be extended through clinical signs of abnormality for which the doctor will search in a physical examination of the patient. The doctor seeks clinical signs through the following processes:

(1) Visual observation (the doctor looks and sees);
(2) Palpation (the doctor touches and feels);
(3) Ausculation (the doctor uses a stethoscope and listens to sound);
(4) Olfaction (the doctor uses the sense of smell);

(5) Percussion (the doctor lightly drums or taps over an underlying structure or a cavity). This percussion yields information through the resonance and pitch of the resultant drumming sound, through vibration which is elicited and through resistance to the tapping which can be felt through the fingers used. The information to be obtained is about the position, the size and the consistency of structures and the presence of fluid in cavities.

In generally observing the patient the doctor (and indeed anyone who has the care of patients at any time) must note the following features:

(1) Level of consciousness;
(2) Colour;
(3) Heartbeat and respiration;
(4) State of skin (dry, moist, hot, cold);
(5) General physical condition.

Fundamental clinical tests

To add to the information which is to be gained from the symptoms which are described and seen, the signs which are sought and the observations which are to be made, there are certain fundamental clinical tests which are undertaken of the patient's body. These are tests of:

(1) The temperature;
(2) The pulse;
(3) The respiration;
(4) The blood pressure.

Elsewhere in this book the reader will find descriptions of how these tests are made, of factors which influence the results and of the possible significance of certain findings. Here it is enough to say that these tests are indeed commonly undertaken both outside hospitals and within them on many patients. All the readers of this book have probably at some time or another undergone at least one of these tests and many may have had all four performed.

These tests involve little in the way of special equipment: a clinical thermometer for the temperature, a sphygmomanometer for the blood pressure and, for the timing, a watch which records seconds. Relatively little training and practice are needed for those who are to carry out the tests.

Special tests and investigations

Moving beyond the four fundamental tests just mentioned, we see ourselves entering an extensive territory, peopled by many different specialists using a great range of methods, substances and items of equipment. We now find ourselves within the hospital contemplating many possibilities for the patient and many facilities to be commanded in search for the diagnosis that must be made if the patient is to be effectively aided.

Since this book is written for radiographers we would emphasize that diagnostic radiology is itself a special test, undertaken by trained staff using refined methods and complex equipment. This is a special test which is carried out on the patient personally in a clinical environment. It is distinct from tests made in laboratories on various specimen substances of one sort or another which in one way or another have been obtained from the patient. The basis of diagnostic radiology is the interpretation by a human observer of a visual image created through the use of X-rays: it is now often considered as one form of diagnostic imaging. There are other forms of clinical diagnostic imaging with which radiographers are currently involved. One is ultrasonography, in which ultrasound waves are used to produce an image for visual interpretation. Another is radionuclide imaging in which certain radiopharmaceuticals (radionuclides which can be given to patients) are used to visualize various organs so that an image is produced for interpretation. A fourth special test in this group designated as diagnostic imaging is a process called magnetic resonance. The basis of the visible image then is information which is obtained through the magnetic properties of atomic nuclei, the atoms concerned being those of various tissues in the human body.

In regard to all the other tests, it seems wise to impose a sense of order by categorizing them according to various systems of the body. Table 16.1 shows the categories and names some tests which are mentioned in the rest of this chapter. Readers must realize that we have omitted a great number of tests, and included only those tests of which radiographers may find some knowledge interesting and even useful as they deal with patients.

Table 16.1 Some special tests used in clinical practice.

Alimentary system	Blood	Cardiovascular system	Respiratory system	Nervous system	Urogenital system
Endoscopy	Blood counts	Blood pressure	Nose and throat swabs	Cerebrospinal fluid	Urine
Liver function	Blood groups	Electrocardiography	Sputum tests		Cystoscopy
Pancreatic efficiency	Rhesus factor		Laryngoscopy		Biopsies
Biopsies			Biopsies		
Tests on faeces			Bronchoscopy		

Note: This table shows only a few tests and omits any testing by means of X-rays or other imaging modalities.

The alimentary tract

Endoscopy (pharynx, oesophagus, stomach, intestines)

The pharynx, oesophagus, stomach and intestines make up a series of linked organs which are hollow spaces or potential spaces. A common special method of investigating the internal aspects of these organs is endoscopy: that is, a visual observation of their insides by means of an endoscope. The endoscope is an instrument comprising a tube and an optical system and the inspection is made by placing the tube inside the organ concerned, by way of either a natural orifice in the body or a small surgical incision. Table 16.2 names organs so investigated, the examinations and the instruments used.

Table 16.2 Endoscopy of the alimentary tract.

The organs	The examinations	The instruments used
Pharynx	Pharyngoscopy	Pharyngoscope
Oesophagus	Oesophagoscopy	Oesophagoscope
Stomach	(1) Gastroscopy	(1) Gastroscope
	(1) Gastric photography	(2) Gastric camera
Duodenum	Duodenoscopy	Duodenoscope
Colon	Colonoscopy	Coloscope
Rectum	Proctoscopy	Proctoscope
Intra-abdominal organs and peritoneal cavity	Laparascopy	Laparoscope (inserted into peritoneal cavity through small incision in anterior abdominal wall)

These methods of visual inspection have a wide range of modern practice through the use of fibreoptic endoscopes. Fibreoptic technology allows light images to be transmitted by glass fibres and its developments have greatly extended the examinations which can be made and the scope of the information which can be gained. The glass fibres are long and flexible and transmit light images round corners. So that endoscopy is now rather more like walking into a room to see what is there and rather less like trying to assess a room by putting one eye to the keyhole of its locked door!

Another development is the gastric camera which is passed into the stomach. This specially designed camera records images on a film which is specially made for the purpose.

Liver function and pancreatic efficiency

One of the functions of the liver is to form bile which is stored in the gall bladder and eventually enters the duodenum when fatty foods are there.

Bile contains bile pigments and bile salts. When there is altered excretion of bile pigments, the bile pigment bilirubin is retained in the blood and if the level rises excessively the patient becomes jaundiced.

Laboratory tests of specimens of blood and urine enable a diagnosis to be made of the type of jaundice which is present. It may be:

(1) Obstructive – due to blocked bile ducts which prevent the bile from entering the duodenum;
(2) Haemolytic – due to excessive breakdown of red blood cells which raises the level of bilirubin in the blood;
(3) Infective – due to the presence of a specific pathogenic micro-organism.

The pancreas produces (1) *digestive enzymes* which are discharged through pancreatic ducts into the duodenum (Evans, 1989); and (2) *the hormone insulin* which is secreted directly into the bloodstream from the special cells of the pancreas known as the islets of Langerhans. Investigation as to the efficiency of the pancreas may be made through laboratory tests of blood, of urine, of fluid from the duodenum, of sweat and of the fat content in the faeces.

Tests of the faeces

Among other tests, the faeces may be examined for the presence of micro-organisms, parasites and blood. Blood which is visible and recognizable by sight in the faeces is called *frank blood*. That it can be seen to be obvious red blood means that it is unchanged by the processes of the digestive tract and the haemorrhage is occurring at a point which is relatively low in the tract or is at the anus. Blood which is not visible to the naked eye is called *occult blood* and its presence can be shown by laboratory tests. The term melaena means that the faeces are black and tarry in appearance. This is due to the presence of altered blood, changed by its processing through the digestive system. This alternation suggests that the point of haemorrhage is high up in the gastrointestinal tract; or that the blood has been swallowed from a bleeding nose, mouth or facial injury.

Tests of the blood

As it circulates through the body the blood carries nourishment, electrolytes, hormones, vitamins, heat, oxygen and antibodies. There are many special examinations which may be made of it and these can be categorized into the following groups:

(1) Tests associated with haematology and blood transfusion;

(2) Tests which are bacteriological;
(3) Tests which are chemical.

Table 16.3 indicates the scope of the tests in these groups but we propose to consider only two of them in more detail than simply their display in the table. These two are *blood counts* and the *determination of blood groupings*.

Table 16.3 Examination of the blood.

Haematology and blood transfusion	Bacteriological tests	Chemical tests
Blood counts	Blood cultures	Level of alcohol
Blood groups	Tests for various specific diseases	Bile pigments
Bone marrow puncture		Salts
Bleeding time		Acids
Clotting time		Cholesterol
		Electrolytes
		Drugs
		Sugar
		Fats
		Urea
		Hormones

Blood counts

The fluid part of the blood is called plasma and 90% of it is water. Suspended in the plasma are:

(1) Red blood corpuscles (erythrocytes);
(2) White blood corpuscles (leucocytes);
(3) Platelets (thrombocytes);
(4) Fat globules;
(5) Many chemical substances, carbohydrates, proteins, hormones, oxygen.

The red corpuscles function to carry oxygen to the body's tissues and to this end they contain haemoglobin: this is a substance which has iron in it and it combines well with oxygen. The white cells are of two main types: granulocytes and agranulocytes. Some of them have a property called phagocytosis. This means that they have the ability to take up foreign matter such as the bodies of pathogenic bacteria and bits of dead tissue. Some of them have a part to play in the formation of antibodies. In general it could be said that the leucocytes are important to the abilities of the body to combat infection and to resolve inflammation and to keep itself free of disease: that is, to maintain immunity. The platelets are important in the normal process of clotting blood in the natural arrest of haemorrhage.

A blood count is a laboratory examination of a specimen of blood which is taken from the patient. A small specimen may be obtained by pricking a fingertip or an earlobe and squeezing forth a drop of blood. A larger amount may be drawn from a vein (in the arm, for example) by means of a hypodermic needle and syringe:

Information is commonly sought about the following:

(1) The level of haemoglobin in the blood as an indication of the oxygen-carrying capacity of the blood;
(2) The number of red cells present;
(3) The appearances of the red cells, that is their size and their colour;
(4) The number of white cells present;
(5) The differential white cell count, this being a statement as to the proportions of the different sorts of white cells which are present.

Tables 16.4 and 16.5 set out some facts and some terminology about blood counts.

Blood groups and blood transfusion

The human population can be categorized into four main blood groups which are of great importance when one person (the recipient) is transfused with blood provided from another (the donor). In the blood serum are found agglutinins: these are antibodies which can make red cells of another's blood clump together – that is, the red cells agglutinate. In the red cells are found agglutinogens: these are antigens with which the serum agglutinins react to produce the clumping (agglutination) of the red cells. The risk in blood transfusion is that the red cells in the donated blood (donor's red cells) will be agglutinated when their red cell agglutinogens and the serum agglutinins of the recipient react together. The donor gives a relatively small volume to the recipient and the red cells of this small volume are subjected to the full volume of the recipient's serum. When the red cells clump they block capillary circulation, toxic products are released and great damage is caused.

In the donor's serum the agglutinins are not likely to have much effect on the red cells of the recipient: the donor serum is diluted by the greater volume of the recipient's blood. So the recipient's red cells are safe from the donated serum. It is the donated red cells which are at risk from the recipient's serum.

The four main blood groups mentioned earlier are grouped according to the agglutinogens which are present in the red cells. The four groups are as shown in Table 16.6, designated A, B, AB, and O. It can be seen that Group

Table 16.4 Blood Counts.

The test	Normal average result	Variations from the normal
Haemoglobin level	14.5 g per decilitre of blood for adult Below 11.5 g/dl is anaemia Above 1800 g/dl is polycythaemia	Anaemia is a state in which the body lacks the normal (a) level of haemoglobin, or (b) number of red blood cells, or (c) level of haemoglobin *and* number of red cells. Polycythaemia is the state when the blood contains more red cells than the normal number and has a higher level of haemoglobin.
Red cell count and red cell appearances	5.00×10^{12} per litre for males 4.5×10^{12} per litre for females	In pernicious anaemia the red cell count and the haemoglobin level are low and a significant sign is that the red cells increase in size and may be nearly twice as large as is normal. In iron deficiency anaemia the red cells are reduced in size but not in number and they are pale in colour. Haemoglobin level is lowered.
White cells count	4.00 to 11.00×10^9 per litre	Leucocytosis is an increase in number above 11.00×10^9. Leucopaenia is a decrease in number below 4.00×10^9. In myeloid leukaemia the white cell count may rise to 50.00×10^9 per litre.
Differential white cell count	Polymorphs 1.5 to 7.5×10^9 per litre Lymphocytes 1.00 to 4.5×10^9 per litre Monocytes up to 0.8×10^9 per litre Eosinophils up to 0.4×10^9 per litre Basophils up to 0.2×10^9 per litre	Polymorphs increase in most acute infections and in sepsis. Lymphocytes and monocytes increase in glandular fever. Eosinophils increase in allergic conditions.
Platelet count	150 to 350×10^9 per litre	Reduction below 40×10^9 per litre is likely to be followed by haemorrhage. A number increased above the normal range predisposes to embolus.

Evans (1989), pp 103 and 109.

Table 16.5 Variations from the normal in blood counts.

Blood component	Level lowered	Level raised
Haemoglobin	The anaemias. Severe haemorrhage. Interference with the normal production of red cells (for example in faulty diet; in some malabsorptions of foodstuffs; in certain neoplasms; in use of certain drugs; after irradiation with ionizing radiation). Excessive destruction of red cells (for example in rhesus incompatibility; in transfusion with incompatible blood; in certain infections).	
Red cells	Severe haemorrhage. The anaemias. Interference with production of or excessive destruction of red cells (see above).	Normal physiological response to high altitude. Heart and lung diseases which interfere with the oxygenation of blood. At birth and for 24 hours following. Small repeated haemorrhages. Slightly after exercise or eating a full meal. Dehydration from any cause. Polycythaemia.
White cells	Typhoid fever. Influenza. Measles. Malaria. Aplastic anaemia. Chronic haemorrhage. Malnutrition. Lead, mercury, arsenic poisoning. Irradiation by ionizing radiation.	The leukaemias. Most acute infections and sepsis. Glandular fever. Allergic conditions. Normal physiological response to great muscular activity. Emotion. Dehydration. Digestion of meals.
Platelets	Aplastic anaemia. Leukaemia. Diseases of bone marrow. Scurvy.	After surgery, especially splenectomy.

Table 16.6 Blood groups.

Group	Agglutinogens in red cells	Agglutinins in serum which are against:
A	A	Agglutinogens B (anti-B)
B	B	Agglutinogens A (anti-A)
AB	A and B	No agglutinins
O	No agglutinogens	Agglutinogens A (anti-A) and agglutinogens B (anti-B)

A has serum agglutinins which will agglutinate Group B red cells; and that Group B has agglutinins (known as anti-A) which will agglutinate Group A red cells. As Group AB has no agglutinins in the serum there will be no agglutination of any donated red cells so Group AB is known as a universal recipient. Group O has in its serum agglutinins which will agglutinate the red cells of Group A and Group B and in Group O red cells there are no agglutinogens. These red cells cannot be agglutinated by the serum agglutinins of any recipient: so Group O is a universal donor. These facts are set out in Table 16.7.

In blood transfusion the preferred course is to transfuse the recipient with blood from a donor who is of the same group. If that is not available in an emergency, the recipient can be given blood from a donor whose red cells

Table 16.7 Blood groups and blood transfusion.

Donor group	Donor cells are agglutinated by recipient group	Safe recipient groups
A	B O	A A B
B	A O	B A B
A B	A B O	A B
O	No recipient group	A B A B O

Note
Group A B appears throughout the *safe recipient* column – is universal recipient.
Group O has no possibility for its cells to be agglutinated by any recipient – is universal donor.

agglutinogens will not react with the recipient's serum agglutinins (see Table 16.7).

In the population of the United Kingdom the four main blood groups are distributed as shown in Fig. 16.1. The more widespread groups are O and A, the groups B and AB being much less frequently found.

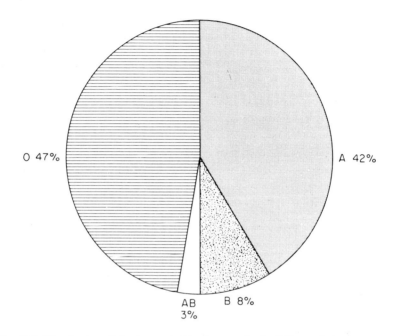

Fig. 16.1 Distribution of the four main blood groups in the UK population.

The rhesus factor

There is another agglutinogen to be found in the red blood corpuscles which is called the rhesus factor because the same agglutinogen is also found in the red cells of rhesus monkeys. Anyone who has this factor present is said to be rhesus positive; 85% of the population is rhesus positive. The remaining 15% do not have this rhesus positive factor in their red blood corpuscles and are said to be rhesus negative (see Fig. 16.2).

The rhesus factor is significant in blood transfusion because if a recipient who is rhesus negative (Rh-negative) is given an injection of blood which is rhesus positive (Rh-positive) the Rh-negative subject can develop serum agglutinins (as a result of this first transfusion) that will agglutinate the red cells in a subsequent donation of Rh-positive blood. So people who are Rh-negative should not be transfused with Rh-positive blood.

This production of serum agglutinins in the Rh-negative subject is of obstetrical significance in women who are Rh-negative. The rhesus factor is

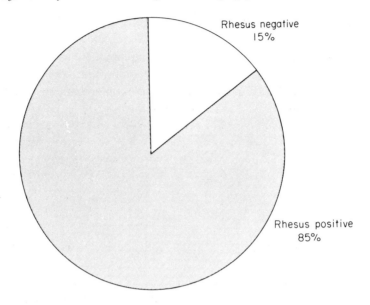

Fig. 16.2 Proportion of rhesus negative individuals in the UK population.

an inherited characteristic and the Rh-negative mother may carry a fetus which has a positive rhesus factor inherited from the Rh-positive father. Through the placenta, the Rh-positive fetal blood may cause the mother to develop agglutinins in her blood serum which (again via the placenta) may agglutinate the red blood cells of the embryo.

This effect may not be marked in a first pregnancy (unless the mother has earlier developed the agglutinins as a result of a blood transfusion with Rh-positive blood) but in subsequent pregnancies the consequences can be very serious. There will be destruction of red blood cells (haemolysis) with results of varying severity:

(1) A still-born baby;
(2) A baby born alive with severe jaundice who may subsequently develop cerebral damage;
(3) A baby born alive with some degree of haemolytic anaemia which is not severe.

A method of treating haemolytic anaemia in the new born is to carry out an exchange transfusion in which the baby's blood is completely replaced with blood of rhesus compatibility.

There is a way of evading the hazard of the rhesus factor. If, within 72 hours of delivery, Rh-negative mothers are injected with gamma G-immunoglobulin they do not develop the agglutinins which agglutinate the Rh-positive blood.

The cardiovascular system

The blood pressure

Essentially the cardiovascular system is one of closed pipes (the blood vessels) within which the blood is circulated by means of a driving pump (the heart). There is a certain more or less constant volume of blood to be circulated and as it goes round it puts pressure on the walls of the vessels (arteries, capillaries, veins). This pressure is the blood pressure. The blood pressure is high in the arteries and highest in the large arteries not far from the heart, which forcefully pumps out a quantity of blood with each contraction (systole). As the blood flows into smaller arteries and eventually to capillaries the pressure becomes less. This falling pressure continues as the blood flows into veins on its return journey to the heart and the pressure is lowest in the large veins close to the heart.

In the arteries the pressure is highest when the heart contracts to pump out blood: this is the systolic pressure. In the phase of relaxation between the systoles the blood pressure is lower (diastolic pressure) and is then about two-thirds of the systolic pressure. The systolic pressure changes with states of physical activity or emotional excitement, whereas the diastolic pressure is relatively constant.

Blood pressure depends on the following.

(1) The volume of blood which is circulating. A decrease in volume (for example after marked loss of blood) results in a fall in pressure. So low blood pressure may be one of the signs of internal haemorrhage.
(2) The viscosity of the blood, this being affected by proteins in the blood plasma and the numbers of blood cells.
(3) The elasticity of the walls of large blood vessels.
(4) The resistance which the walls of peripheral vessels offer (peripheral resistance) to the blood as it goes along them. This increases if the vessels are constricted or narrowed.

The level of the blood pressure is influenced by the patient's posture and emotional state. Blood pressure is lowest in sleep and highest in the first circumstances of the erect posture and the disturbed state.

Hypertension is the term used for blood pressures which are above the normal range. *Hypotension* means that the blood pressure is below the normal range.

There are several diseases and states in which one of the signs may be altered blood pressure. For example, blood pressure falls in shock, in haemorrhage and in fainting attacks. Blood pressure rises in some forms of nephritis (a group of diseases affecting the kidneys), in some diseases of the renal arteries and in raised intracranial pressure from a head injury or a brain tumour.

When the pathological state is corrected by treatment, the blood pressure may be rectified also because the changed pressure is secondary to a known cause which is the diseased state present. In contrast to this there is a condition called *essential hypertension* in which the patient has a blood pressure which is higher than normal and the cause is not known: it is primary and not a secondary state. In about 90% of the patients who present themselves to a doctor with blood pressure above normal the hypertension is of unknown origin.

Electrocardiography

Electrocardiography is the recording of the electrical activity of the heart during the course of the cardiac cycle. The cycle comprises contraction of the two atria while the ventricles relax, followed by contraction of the ventricles with relaxation of the atria and then a pause. The initiation of the cardiac cycle and the control for the co-ordination of events come from within the heart muscle itself: there are specialized areas of cells in the heart muscle which carry out these functions and this special tissue may be called the pacemaker of the heart. Many people nowadays are aware of the possibility of inserting an artificial pacemaker which is an electrical device to control the beating heart if the natural pacemaker is faulty.

Whether naturally or artificially controlled, the cardiac cycle of events is accompanied by electrical changes. An electrocardiogram is a record of these changes displayed in the form of a graph. The graph may be recorded as a tracing on special paper, in which case a permanent record is provided. Or the graph may be a continuous dynamic display on an electrocardiograph (ECG) monitor or cardiac oscilloscope such as is used in an intensive therapy unit (ITU) for the immediate detection of abnormal rhythms (cardiac arrhythmias) and of abnormal rates of the heartbeat.

The graph of the heart's activity is a wavy line which usually shows recognizable points in the cardiac cycle of events. Fig. 16.3 shows typical patterns in normal electrocardiographs. ECG monitoring can be done as an integral part of certain X-ray examinations, e.g. cardioangiography.

The electrocardiogram provides significant information about the heart-rate and the rhythms of the heart and the state of the heart muscle. Below are some terms which the student will encounter relating to the heart.

Bradycardia	Abnormally slow rate of beat.
Tachycardia	Abnormally fast rate of beat.
Fibrillation	Very rapid incomplete contractions which are
(atrial or ventricular)	irregular, unco-ordinated and ineffectual.

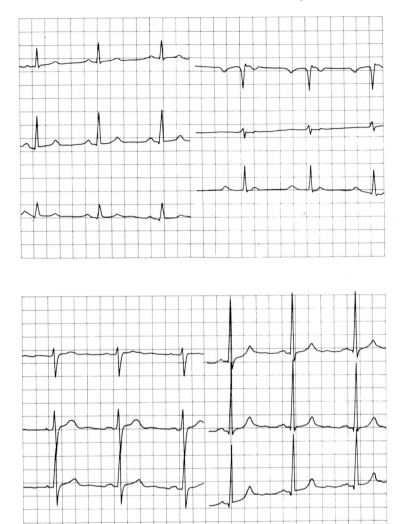

Fig. 16.3 Typical normal electrocardiograph patterns.

Extrasystoles	Premature contractions which happen in addition to the basic rhythm of the heartbeat.
Heart block	Failure of the conducting tissue of the heart (the pacemaker) to conduct impulses for contraction normally from the atria to the ventricles: heart block may be incomplete, giving a conducting-time which is longer than the normal one, or it may be complete, with the result that the atrial and ventricular contractions are completely dissociated from each other.

The respiratory system

Parts of the respiratory tract are accessible to visual inspection by means of endoscopes: that is, by means of special instruments with optical systems which can be used for looking at the interiors of organs and cavities. Table 16.8 shows the range of examinations and instruments.

Table 16.8 Endoscopy of the respiratory tract.

The organs	The examinations	The instruments
Nose	Rhinoscopy	Rhinoscope
Pharynx	Pharyngoscopy	Pharyngoscope
Larynx	Laryngoscopy	Laryngoscope
Trachea and main bronchi	Bronchoscopy	Bronchoscope

Other tests of the respiratory tract are laboratory tests made on sputum. These may show the presence of the following: blood; pus; fibrous tissue from destruction of lungs; micro-organisms. Other laboratory tests may be made on material (tissue, secretions) which is collected from the nose or throat by wiping the area with a swab, the swab being made of cotton or gauze which is on the end of a thin stick so that it may be applied to the part concerned. The matter gained by swabbing can be tested for the presence of micro-organisms.

The nervous system

Among the multitude of tests which may be made of the nervous system, we mention here just one: that is, the examination of cerebrospinal fluid (CSF). Cerebrospinal fluid is a thin water-like fluid of exceptional clarity which forms in the ventricular system of the brain and circulates from there to the subarachnoid space. This space is between two of the three membranes (dura mater, arachnoid mater, pia mater) which entirely surround the brain and spinal cord. The cerebrospinal fluid is eventually absorbed into the bloodstream. Its functions are not fully known but it is believed to be involved in the metabolism of nutrients, the removal of waste and the protection of the brain and spinal cord by keeping them (as it does) floating in fluid which is a shock-absorber.

A specimen (for example, 5 ml) of cerebrospinal fluid is obtained by aspiration: that is, through drawing the fluid by suction up a special needle into a syringe. The procedure is strictly sterile in the conditions of its undertaking.

The needle is commonly inserted into the subarachnoid space in the lumbar region of the spine at the level which is between the fourth and fifth lumbar vertebrae. This is to keep it below the level where the spinal cord terminates at a point between the first and second lumbar vertebrae. The process is called a lumbar puncture and the needle is a lumbar puncture needle. Sometimes a lumbar approach is not used and a cisternal puncture is made. In this procedure, the needle is placed into the cisterna magna at a point of insertion between the occipital bone and the first cervical vertebra: the cisterna magna is that part of the subarachnoid space which is immediately below the brain and above the foramen magnum of the occipital bone.

However the specimen is obtained, examined of the cerebrospinal fluid may be helpful as follows:

(1) Colour – a yellow tinge suggests the presence of blood;
(2) Presence of blood – indicates subarachnoid haemorrhage;
(3) Coagulation on standing – indications of meningitis;
(4) Cells present – identification of specific conditions;
(5) Bacteria present – identification of specific infecting organisms.

The urinary system

Clinical tests relating to the urinary system might be said to begin at their simplest with tests that can be carried out on specimens of urine in wards and clinics and even by the patient themselves (after some instruction) in their own home. These tests are easy to perform and interpret since they rest on ordinary visual observation and on the use of special test-papers which are placed in the sample of urine and watched for changes of colours in the papers. In regard to examining the urine, the following are to be considered:

(1) Colour of urine;
(2) Clarity or its opposite turbidity;
(3) Volume of urine passed;
(4) Presence of blood;
(5) Specific gravity of urine;
(6) Presence of abnormal constituents (proteins, sugar);
(7) pH value (acidity/alkalinity).

Taken from the clinic to the laboratory, the urine can be tested further for blood, pus, specific infective organisms, abnormal constituents, amounts of normal constituents. More extensive tests can provide information as to the efficiency with which the kidneys are carrying out their functions in (1) the excretion of waste products; and (2) maintaining the normal balance of water and electrolytes in the body's fluids (Evans, 1989 pp. 192–212).

The interiors of the bladder and the urethra may be examined by visual inspection as shown in Table 16.9.

Table 16.9 Endoscopy of the bladder and urethra.

The organs	The examinations	The instruments
Bladder	Cystoscopy	Cystoscope
Urethra	Urethroscopy	Panendoscope

Biopsy

Biopsy is a surgical procedure in which a small piece of tissue is taken from the patient for the purpose of sending it for microscopic examination in a laboratory. The aim of the examination is diagnostic, directed towards identifying the lesions which may be present and it is especially useful in determining the malignancy or innocence of a neoplasm.

There are many tissues of the body which are accessible for biopsy. The tissue may be removed under anaesthesia which is local or general according to the site from which it is being taken and the method which is used. Table 16.10 explains some biopsies which may be performed. The radiographer must remember that all such examinations are traumatic for the patient as they present to the patient the possibility that he/she may have cancer and that the examination may be a prelude to radical treatment and further, possibly disfiguring, surgery. It is important to bear such considerations in mind and to remember the psychological care of the patient as well as the need for physical diagnosis.

Reference

Evans, D.M.D. (1989) Special Tests: *The Procedure and Meaning of the Commoner Tests in Hospital*, (pages 103, 109, 168–9, 192–212), 13th Edn. Mosby Year Book Europe Ltd.

Table 16.10 Biopsies.

Site	Method
Bladder	Biopsy carried out during cystoscopy.
Bone marrow	Superficial bone (sternum, ilium) is penetrated by means of a special instrument and a small specimen of bone marrow is removed from the cavity.
Breast	Carried out by fine needle aspiration (sometimes as part of a mammographic examination) or, under a surgical anaesthetic, a larger excision of tissue may be carried out ('lumpectomy').
Bronchi	Biopsy carried out during bronchoscopy.
Cervix uteri	Cervical cytology (study of cells) is a method of investigation in which smears are taken from the cervix of the uterus and the cells are microscopically examined for the presence of a malignancy in its pre-invasive stage (it is not growing and invading tissue). If the smear-test is positive, cone biopsy confirms the diagnosis.
Colon	Biopsy can be carried out during colonoscopy.
Kidney	After a urogram to establish the position of the kidneys, a renal puncture needle is used for the biopsy. A small specimen of tissue is drawn up (aspiration biopsy) from the kidney through the needle which is inserted at a selected point through the abdominal wall from the outside.
Liver	Aspiration biopsy by means of a biopsy needle which is passed directly into the liver, entering through the abdominal wall at a chosen site over the liver.
Mouth	Biopsy is carried out through direct viewing into the open mouth.
Rectum	Biopsy can be undertaken during proctoscopy.
Small intestine	Biopsy can be performed by means of a Crosby capsule, a small hollow capsule which the patient swallows. The capsule holds a guarded spring-loaded cutting edge which is actuated by a flexible wire which extends from the capsule and remains outside after the patient has swallowed the capsule. Radiographs are taken to check the position of the capsule and at the appropriate point the biopsy is performed by actuating the knife-edge. The capsule contains the small specimen of tissue when it is withdrawn.
Spleen	Aspiration biopsy is performed by means of a biopsy needle inserted directly into the spleen through a selected point on the abdominal wall.
Stomach	Biopsy can be performed during gastroscopy.

Chapter 17
First Aid in the X-ray Department

First aid is the immediate treatment given to a patient by those who are present when an emergency condition arises. While working in the X-ray department, radiographers may be required to help patients in various states that need immediate treatment or immediate assistance. It is clear that certain first aid procedures (for example, treatment of victims rescued from drowning or found with gas poisoning) are *not* likely to be used in the X-ray department. There are, however, several conditions which will be quite commonly encountered (for example, faintness, nausea) and knowledge of what to do for the patient in these circumstances is certainly necessary to a radiographer. Since accidents may happen in spite of every precaution, simple principles of first aid for certain types of accident should also be known.

The objectives of the first aider are:

(1) To save life;
(2) To prevent a worsening condition;
(3) To promote recovery.

The responsibilities of the first aider are:

(1) To assess the situation and identify the state of the patient;
(2) To give suitable first aid treatment at once and to treat first the most urgent conditions;
(3) To appreciate that the most urgent life-threatening states that require treatment at once are cardiac arrests; respiratory arrest; asphyxia; severe haemorrhage;
(4) To arrange for the patient to be properly transferred to medical or nursing care as appropriate (Marsden *et al.* 1992).

It should be taken as a general rule by student radiographers that immediate seniors should be informed and fetched to the scene if something untoward happens to a patient who may be alone with the student, even if the incident appears to be transient in its effect. This does *not* mean that the patient should be abandoned while others are fetched. The student should stay with the patient to give such immediate aid as may be required, if necessary calling out to attract the attention of others, or using a panic button, if available. The student should *not* transmit to the patient a sense of anxiety, but should certainly report to seniors anything about a patient which gives cause for anxiety, though it may seem trivial.

Even if no medical assistance has been required at the time, it will be usual for the radiographer to report further what has happened – in some cases to the radiologist, in others to the ward staff or to the medical officer who referred the patient for X-ray examination. In the event of an accident in the department a full report must be made in writing at the time.

Radiological emergencies

The term *radiological emergency* has come to be associated in particular with a dangerous condition arising in a patient as the result of the use of a radiological contrast agent (see also Chapter 7). However, an emergency may be precipitated not necessarily by this but by some other cause, for example, the administration of a local anaesthetic, pre-existent cardiovascular disease, or even an accident such as electric shock.

Depending on the cause, details of the treatment naturally will vary but the several treatments of serious emergencies overlap to a large extent. The professional responsibility of the radiographer does not extend to decisions about medical treatment. This section will be concerned only with those measures of immediate aid with which every radiographer should be conversant. It is upon the rapidity with which appropriate action can be taken by the person nearest at hand that the patient's life may depend; the nearest person is quite likely to be the radiographer making the X-ray examination or even a senior student who is assisting at it.

In any medical emergency of this kind, as has been said, the radiographer or student must at once call or send for medical assistance. X-ray rooms should be provided with an alarm system so that the radiographer may easily obtain help without having to leave the patient. The two most urgent situations are *cardiac arrest* (cessation of the heartbeat) and *respiratory arrest* (failure to breathe), and these are discussed below.

Cardiac and respiratory arrest

A patient whose brain is deprived of oxygenated blood for longer than 3–4 minutes is likely to suffer irreversible cerebral damage. It is consequently of supreme importance that the diagnosis of cardiac arrest be made quickly and treatment be begun quickly. Cardiac arrest cannot be treated on its own, since it will be accompanied by respiratory failure; restored cerebral circulation is of no use to the patient if the blood is inadequately oxygenated.

In a patient who appears to have collapsed the signs of cardiac arrest are:

(1) Absence of a palpable arterial pulse (carotid artery in the neck);
(2) Dilation of the pupils (a late sign, not seen within 1 minute);
(3) Pallor or cyanosis;
(4) Convulsions (these occur sometimes as a secondary manifestation of diminished cardiac output).

The above observations should be made within 20–30 seconds of the onset of symptoms. In the list, (2) and (4) can occur from other causes. Absence of the arterial pulse is of decisive significance and the radiographer must not hesitate to look for it while awaiting the arrival of medical aid. In the present emergency the pulse may be palpated at any convenient point related to a large artery in the body. However, the carotid artery is perhaps the one of choice since it can be felt in either side of the neck relatively easily by the inexperienced. The two first fingers of one hand should be used to palpate the artery at the anterior border of the sternomastoid muscle, level with the upper edge of the thyroid cartilage (colloquially the 'Adam's apple'). In a small child, the brachial pulse is easier to palpate than the carotid. This is palpated at the elbow where the brachial artery may be felt along the medial side of the biceps brachii muscle (Tortora & Anagnostakos, 1990, p 620).

If cardiac arrest is thought to have occurred, or even is suspected, the single-handed operator has to face the problem of whether to tackle first the cardiac or respiratory failure. The first and most important thing to do, however, is to call for the cardiac arrest team. The priorities for proceeding are then as follows:

A – airway
B – breathing
C – circulation.

A – airway

A simple finger sweep is adopted to ensure that there is no debris blocking the patient's airway. The airway should be opened up by placing a hand on the patient's forehead to tilt the head back and the other hand under the chin to pull the mandible forward. This action lifts the tongue away from the pharyngeal wall and the epiglottis from the laryngeal inlet, thus ensuring a clear airway. This is always the priority in treatment. Great care needs to be taken, however, not to over-tilt the head if there is any suggestion of a spinal cord injury (Coady, 1994).

B – breathing

The blood may be oxygenated by pulmonary ventilation. Deep inhalations provide exhalations which are of use to the patient and can maintain the oxygen tension in his arterial blood nearly at its normal level. The carbon dioxide present in the exhaled breath has a useful function in stimulating the respiratory centre of the brain.

Should the operator who has to continue the procedure for long become dizzy or feel himself grow faint he is suffering from the effects of over-ventilation and has probably been breathing too fast; he should decrease his rate in this event. Like most methods of artificial respiration, expired air resuscitation is tiring but should not otherwise cause physical disturbance. It is often said that the main objection to it is an aesthetic revulsion from mouth-to-mouth contact with a stranger. However, nice considerations of hygiene can hardly be of much weight when the patient is in such an extreme condition.

The procedure can be made to seem more hygienic and acceptable if an airway is available and can be inserted; this may be impossible if the jaw is tightly closed.

Pulmonary ventilation

The term *pulmonary ventilation* refers to the simple processes by which it is sought to re-oxygenate the lungs of a patient who is in respiratory failure. These are:

(1) Artificial respiration;
(2) The supplementary administration of oxygen.

A number of means of performing artificial respiration are known and have been used to good effect. However, at present the method most widely advocated is the one which is known properly as *expired air resuscitation* and popularly in magazines and newspapers as 'the kiss of life'.

Expired air resuscitation

The essence of this procedure is that the operator employs their own exhaled breath to inflate the lungs of the patient. This is done by placing the mouth either directly upon the patient's mouth, or to an airway in the patient's mouth, or sometimes to the patient's nose, the mouth being kept closed; in the case of a small child the mouth and nose can be entered simultaneously.

For the same of simplicity the procedure will be described below as direct mouth-to-mouth respiration. Its steps are as follows.

(1) Make sure by swabbing the patient's mouth that no foreign material is present which may prevent breathing, particularly if there has been vomiting (AIRWAY).

(2) Maintain a clear airway by pulling the patient's jaw upwards. Keep the head tilted back.
(3) Catch the patient's nostrils firmly between the flexed index and middle fingers of your right hand to prevent any escape of air by this route.
(4) Take a deep breath.
(5) Open your mouth wide and place it tightly over both the patient's mouth and your own thumb. It is important to ensure a good seal (see Fig. 17.1).
(6) Exhale – forcibly if the patient is an adult, in a gentle puff in the case of a small child.
(7) The patient's chest should be seen to rise. If it does not do so, suspect the presence of an obstruction and check this possibility again.
(8) Remove your mouth to allow the patient to exhale (which should happen at first passively owing to the elastic recoil of the lungs), and yourself to take a fresh breath. Repeat from (4), continuing at the rate of one inflation every 5 seconds, until the patient is breathing naturally.

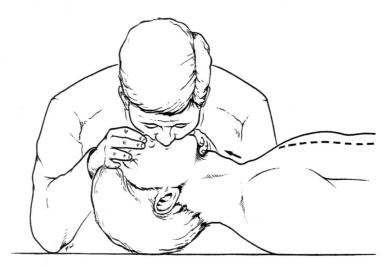

Fig. 17.1 Direct mouth-to-mouth expired air resuscitation. *(Reproduced by courtesy of the Medical Art Department, The Royal Marsden NHS Trust.)*

This method of artificial respiration needs little practice and little knowledge for successful use. It can be employed rapidly on the onset of respiratory emergency, since it does not require the patient to be moved, as do some other methods, into a special position which might necessitate their being taken off the X-ray table. It can be applied instantly by a radiographer alone with the patient. It can do no possible harm if it is begun by someone who believes, but is not absolutely certain, that the patient is lifeless.

The operator should take deep breaths, equivalent to about twice his normal tidal volume. The oxygen content of expired air is naturally lower than atmospheric air, being about 14–18% as against 21%.

C – circulation

External chest compression

External chest compression is performed by means of rhythmic manual compression of the sternum. For it to be successful the patient must be supine upon a *hard* surface. The floor or the X-ray table is suitable but a patient on a mattress should be moved to the floor, or a board or similar structure, for example a large cassette, should be placed at the back of the thorax. The operator should make certain that the patient has a clear airway; the head should be tilted back.

To perform external cardiac massage the operator should take up a position on the patient's right and place the heel of the right hand over the lower sternum; the other hand is superimposed on its fellow with the heels of both hands directly on top of one another and the fingers interlocked (see Fig. 17.2). Pressure is applied vertically downwards 80 times per minute. The operator should be in a position to make use of their body weight for each thrust – that is, their arms should be stiffened – and the sternum should move 4–5 cm towards the vertebral column at every compression. The flaccid condition of the chest wall makes effective movement of the sternum relatively easy to attain. Between compressions the hands should be lifted slightly to permit the chest to expand. Excessive pressure should be avoided. If the operator is a male adult it is probable that external cardiac

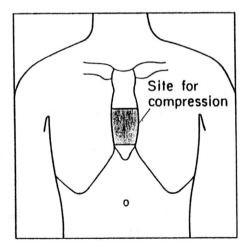

Fig. 17.2 Position of the hands for external chest compression. *(Reproduced by courtesy of the British Journal of Radiology.)*

massage can be efficiently performed with the use of the right hand only, unless the patient is large and the chest unusually rigid. In children up to 10 years of age the force of the heel of one hand is always sufficient; in neonatal infants probably no more than pressure from the fingers alone is required. Since in a young child the heart is relatively higher in the chest, the pressure should be applied over the mid-sternum. Circulation may be deemed adequate if the pupils are contracted.

In the performance of external cardiac massage it is important to remember that the pressure should be applied *only* to the sternum: otherwise rib fractures, haemothorax and liver lacerations have been known to occur. The occurrence of extensive rib fractures necessarily diminishes the efficacy of the performance which depends partly on a general increase in the intrathoracic pressure.

The sequence of cardiopulmonary resuscitation (CPR)

If the patient is not breathing and does not have a pulse then pulmonary ventilation must be combined with external chest compression. Resuscitation attempts **must** be continued until either a pulse returns or the cardiac arrest team arrives and takes over.

If you are alone then commence by giving two breaths of artificial ventilation followed by 15 chest compressions. This sequence should be repeated until help arrives. If there are two people, then once help has been summoned one person should undertake ventilation whilst the other performs chest compression; one breath of ventilation should be given after every five compressions (Marsden *et al.*, 1992, p 38).

Administration of oxygen

Oxygen administered by a face mask is helpful treatment in all instances of radiological emergency. The procedure is detailed in Chapter 9 under the heading Oxygen therapy. If available, a mechanical resuscitator such as a bag and mask is more effective than expired air resuscitation, but you **must** be practised in their operation before attempting to use such equipment on a patient.

It is advisable to have certain other equipment available within easy reach for use when the first stage of emergency has been weathered. This need not be maintained in the X-ray room but will be available in an accessible place somewhere in the department and clearly labelled as an emergency box. These kits are regularly checked and usually contain such equipment as:

● Bag/mask apparatus;
● Mouth gag;

- Laryngoscope;
- Sphygmomanometer and stethoscope;
- Tracheostomy set and certain emergency drugs.

The cardiac arrest team will also have their own accessory equipment which they will bring with them.

This accessory equipment should include an ECG machine and an instrument known as a defibrillator. The first of these is an apparatus for visualizing and recording the heart's beat in the form of electrical impulses and tracings (electrocardiographs). The defibrillator also is an electrical instrument. Fibrillation is an abnormal twitching rhythm of the heart: isolated segments of its muscle contract, out of concert with each other. The condition is not self-correcting and death will occur unless defibrillation is performed rapidly. This condition may be corrected by the influence of an electrical shock. The machine is used to administer a single shock or a series of rapid electric shocks to the cardiac muscle which result in a momentary absence of systole. The heart is restarted under the control of a pacemaker which initiates a normal co-ordinated rhythm of contraction.

Abdominal thrust (the Heimlich manoeuvre)

If, in attempting to clear the patient's airway, there appears to be an obstruction in the trachea itself then the abdominal thrust is a technique which can be life-saving. The indications of an obstruction are that there may be difficulty in breathing (dyspnoea) and possible cyanosis, particularly around the lips. The aim of the manoeuvre, therefore, is to remove the obstruction and restore normal breathing.

The first stage is to lean the patient forwards and to administer sharp blows to the back, midway between the shoulder-blades. If this does not appear to be successful then the patient should be stood up. Position yourself behind them with your arms circling the patient's ribcage and your fingers interlocked in the midline at a point just below the ribs. The hands should then be pulled sharply upwards and inwards. This has the effect of compressing the diaphragm and forcibly expelling air from the lungs. This dual effect forces expulsion of air from the trachea and, hopefully with it, the foreign body.

If the first thrust is unsuccessful in removing the obstruction then the manoeuvre should be repeated several times more; interspersing with back blows if necessary. If the patient is unconscious this procedure may be undertaken with the patient supine on the floor. Your should then kneel astride the patient and perform abdominal thrusts with the heels of the hands (Marsden *et al.*, 1992).

Shock

This state is a recognizable condition in patients after injury. It is particularly liable to occur when there has been loss of blood or plasma. The blood loss may not be apparent as visible haemorrhage. For example, a fracture of the femur may result in a loss of 20–30% of the total blood volume into the soft tissues of the thigh. Extensive burns give rise to severe loss of plasma.

While shock is more likely to follow a severe injury, patients show variation due to differences in age, general physical constitution, and temperament, and the degree of shock which will follow any given injury is not predictable, though its likelihood can be foreseen. The physical injury may seem relatively trivial, for the condition of shock may be produced by mental forces acting on physical processes, and can follow from fright and alarm as well as other emotionally disturbing experiences. It is, however, generally agreed that the most important cause of shock is loss of whole blood or plasma from the circulation. Shock can be immediate or delayed, and can vary in degree from slight shock to a condition which is fatal.

The general picture presented by the patient is due to the fact that their body is without a full volume of circulating blood, indicating a general depression of bodily functions in which the blood vessels are more flaccid than they should normally be and the heart beat has lost force.

The patient has lowered blood pressure. His pulse is rapid as the heartbeat increases its rate in an effort to make more blood circulate and provide the patient with more oxygen. At the same time the force of the pulse feels weak. The patient is pale and cold, and he may be sweating or restless. His breathing may be shallow and slow, or it may be sighing in character.

The general treatment is to keep the patient lying down at rest so far as is possible, and to provide some degree of warmth without overheating. The head should be kept low and turned on one side unless there is injury to the head, chest, and abdomen. The legs should be raised and supported to improve blood flow.

A patient who has vomited or seems breathless should be placed immediately in the recovery position – halfway between lying on his side and lying face downwards (see Fig. 11.4 – provided that there are no injuries.

The radiographer will see many patients in a condition of shock while carrying out X-ray examinations on those who have been injured. These general procedures of treatment indicate how such patients should be handled. The patient should not be put erect, or be uncovered more, or for a longer period, than is necessary for the purposes of the X-ray examination.

If the patient collapses to the point of cardiac/respiratory arrest, resuscitation procedures must begin immediately.

Haemorrhage

Haemorrhage may be bleeding from a visible site, known as external haemorrhage, or it may be bleeding which takes place internally. In this case it may be revealed by escape of blood from a natural body orifice.

External haemorrhage

Haemorrhage may be (1) arterial, (2) venous, and (3) capillary. When the bleeding takes place from an external wound the type of haemorrhage can be recognized by the colour of the blood and the way in which it escapes.

Arterial haemorrhage produces bright red blood issuing in spurts which may be of considerable force if a large artery has been damaged. *Venous haemorrhage* causes a steady flow of darker blood. If a large vein is damaged there is a rapid flow of blood, but this type of bleeding is easier to control than that which comes from arteries, when there is much greater pressure behind it. *Capillary haemorrhage* produces a general oozing which is not difficult to control. Blood loss from capillary haemorrhage is generally negligible.

Nature stops the bleeding first of all by contraction of severed vessel walls, secondly by clotting of the blood, and thirdly by lowering of the pressure of the blood within the vessel walls.

A patient who has lost a lot of blood shows paleness of skin and lips. As the reduced amount of blood is unable to carry sufficient oxygen, the body attempts to compensate for this by an increase in the rate at which it is pumped round the heart; although more rapid, the pulse feels weak in force. The patient may breathe with deep and long aspirations because of the need for more oxygen. There is a decrease in the body temperature because of the fluid loss, and skin is cold and clammy. The patient is restless, anxious, thirsty, and feels faint.

The first aid treatment for haemorrhage is directed towards its arrest. If the haemorrhage is external, the first action should be to apply pressure to the wound, if possible with a clean, firm pad. It may, however, be more important to apply the pressure as quickly as possible (for example if the bleeding is arterial and profuse), and in that case the radiographer's thumbs should be pressed on the wound. Firm pressure should be maintained.

In order to aid lowering of the blood pressure, the patient should be put lying flat, with head lowered if possible, unless the bleeding is from head or neck. If the site of haemorrhage is a limb, the limb should be elevated unless there is suspicion of a fracture. Medical assistance should be sought, and the patient should be reassured. It is generally recommended that the patient should be kept warm, but overheating is to be avoided.

It may be presumed that in the X-ray department medical assistance will be available before much time has passed, and it is unlikely that the radiographer will have to maintain for long unaided first aid measures for haemorrhage. The direct pressure on the wound and the general procedures described are probably all that will be required.

If it is not possible to apply direct pressure successfully, indirect pressure may be tried at a point between the wound and the heart. The artery is compressed where it is superficial and lies over a bone against which it can be firmly pressed. *Such pressure should not be maintained for longer than 10 minutes.*

For example, the pressure point for the brachial artery is against the inner side of the humerus about halfway between the medial epicondyle and axilla, the pressure being directed posterolaterally. The inner seam of a coat sleeve is in a position which approximately indicates the course of this artery.

The radial artery is compressible against the distal edge of the radius at the anterior aspect of the wrist joint.

Indirect pressure for the femoral artery is against the bony pelvis at a point where the vessel enters the thigh midway between the symphysis pubis and the anterior superior iliac spine – that is the centre of the groin.

Revealed internal haemorrhage

Emergencies may arise in the X-ray department when patients have a haemorrhage as a result of disease processes in the body. The patient may, for example, vomit blood from the alimentary tract, or cough blood from the lungs. The vomiting of blood is called *haematemesis*; the coughing of blood is called *haemoptysis*. Vomited blood is dark in colour, and blood from the lungs is bright red and frothy, readily distinguished from blood which is vomited.

Clearly there can be no question of applying pressure in either of these conditions, since there is no external wound. The first aid measures are the general ones previously described to be undertaken while medical advice is obtained.

The patient should be reassured and kept at rest as comfortably as possible in a place of privacy, even if the privacy can be only that provided by a screen placed round him. If he is continuing to vomit or cough, he should be assisted in this. The radiographer should provide a bowl and hold it for him, and wipe his mouth every so often with a clean tissue. He will find it easier if he can be supported sitting up, but if this is impossible (he may be too ill to attempt it), then he will have to be positioned and supported lying down with his head turned to one side. The best type of bowl to use is a kidney shaped receiver, as the concavity of the curve fits under the patient's chin and makes a more efficient arrangement. All vomited material should be saved for medical inspection.

Bleeding from the nose (epistaxis)

The patient should be supported sitting up with his head held forward, and he should be told to breathe through his mouth. Direct pressure is easily applied by compressing the nose firmly between finger and thumb at a point just below the bridge. This is likely to be the most effectual way to arrest the haemorrhage in a young subject, when the bleeding is often from a point inside the nostril on the septum of the nose. If the bleeding is persistent and severe, medical advice should be sought. Compression should initially be applied for 10 minutes, then for a further 10 minutes if the bleeding has not stopped.

In an elderly person the bleeding may be from within the bony part of the nose, and thus the point of haemorrhage cannot be compressed. The patient should lie flat with his face turned downwards, and he should be given a bowl into which the blood and saliva may flow. He should be told to breathe through his mouth and not to swallow. If the bleeding is persistent and severe, medical advice must be sought.

Burns and scalds

These two are grouped together for both are injuries produced by heat, the *burn* by dry heat and the *scald* by moist heat. First aid treatment is the same for both conditions. The important features to appreciate with regard to this type of injury are (1) that it can be serious even though superficial in character if a large enough skin area is involved; (2) the degree of pain and shock which will accompany an extensive burn, for such burns even if superficial result in loss of plasma; (3) the danger of infection and sepsis, to which burns are particularly liable.

The best action to take *first* is to immerse the burnt area as soon as possible in cold water. This lowers the temperature of involved tissues and reduces damage. The affected part should be kept in the water until the heat and pain have decreased. The immersion should be for a minimum of 10 minutes. The burnt area should then be covered as soon as possible with a dry dressing, preferably a sterile one; if not sterile, the dressing material must be clean. It should be material with a smooth surface so that there is no fluffiness or roughness of texture to stick to the burned part. If the area is large, sterile or clean dressing towels may be used. Clothing which covers the injury is best left as it is, and should not be cut and pulled away if it is burned on to the skin. In the case of a scald, if the clothing is soaked with boiling water it should obviously be removed.

The extent of the treatment required depends on the severity of the injury. Burns may be classified as superficial, partial thickness or full thickness. Superficial burns involve only the epidermis or outer layer of the skin. Prompt treatment and covering with a sterile dressing is all that is required and such burns usually heal well. Partial thickness burns involve epidermal tissue with some destruction of the dermal layer also. Full thickness burns involve extensive destruction of the dermis and nerve endings and other deep structures are damaged or destroyed. Both partial- and full-thickness burns require medical attention. Badly burned patients may be in great pain and the onset of shock is fairly quick and must be watched for. The degree of shock suffered by any individual patient is determined by the depth and extent of the burns. Wallace's Rule of Nines divides the body's surface into areas of approximately 9% (e.g. arm, front of leg, etc) in order that the extent of a burn may be calculated. Partial thickness burns which affect more than 50% of an adult's body surface can be fatal. The percentage is less in children and elderly patients (Marsden *et al.*, 1992).

Loss of consciousness

The causes of loss of consciousness are various. The state may be partial or it may be complete and different levels of consciousness can be recognized as follows.

(1) The patient is *fully conscious*, aware of the surroundings and able to reply to questions and engage in conversation.
(2) The patient is *drowsy*. They are able to answer direct questions and obey commands but respond vaguely when addressed.
(3) The patient is in a *stupor*. They respond to the stimulus of pain. They appear unaware of surroundings and make no response when addressed.
(4) The patient is *completely unconscious* and makes no response even to painful stimuli.

If you are called upon to give aid to a patient who becomes unconscious while in your department, you need to decide the cause of the loss of consciousness in order to identify the situation with which you are dealing. So here are questions to be asked.

(1) Was the onset gradual or sudden? Was it silent or preceded by a warning of any sort? Was there any incident or is there the presence of a known condition which explains it? Is there visible injury?

(2) What is the level of consciousness?

(3) Is the patient pale, flushed or cyanosed? Is the skin dry or moist, hot or cold?

(4) Is the pulse beat present? Is it slow or fast, weak or strong, regular or irregular?

(5) Are the respirations normal? Regular or irregular, fast or slow, shallow or deep, silent or noisy? Is there any smell on the breath?

(6) Are the limbs and body slack, or rigid? Are there spasmodic muscular contractions?

(7) Is there incontinence of urine or faeces?

General care

Apart from any specialist care required for an unconscious patient and any special procedures which may be needed to treat specific conditions, certain general rules for the care of such patients can be enumerated as below.

(1) Do not leave the patient alone.

(2) See that the patient has a maintained clear airway.

(3) Observe the patient, checking for colour and state of skin, cyanosis, pulse rate and volume and regularity, respiration, level of consciousness.

(4) Be alert for signs of change and begin resuscitation if the patient has cardiac/respiratory arrest.

(5) If the patient recovers consciousness, reassure and help them and maintain your observations while they are in your care.

Fainting attack

The simplest cause of loss of consciousness is a fainting attack; this is due to a temporarily impaired supply of blood to the brain. The condition may arise through emotional causes such as fear or receipt of bad news, or through physical stress such as being in a stuffy room, or in want of food, or in a fatigued state.

The patient looks pale and is sweating visibly on the forehead and about the mouth. They may complain of feeling dizzy, nauseated, or faint, for the loss of consciousness is not sudden. At this stage it may be prevented if the patient lies flat, on the floor if necessary.

If this assistance is to succeed in preventing loss of consciousness, it must be given at once as soon as it is recognized that the patient is feeling faint.

Sometimes it will not be realized that the patient is feeling faint, and the first intimation that something is wrong will be the person's loss of consciousness. This could easily occur, for instance, in the screening room where concentration upon the fluoroscopic technique makes it difficult to maintain steady observation of the patient. If they have lost consciousness, they should be allowed to lie flat where they are (unless it is a position of danger). Tight clothing should be loosened. A plentiful supply of fresh air will help.

Usually patients recover from a simple fainting attack quite quickly. Afterwards the patient should rest for a while, and may be given hot tea or coffee or a drink of water. Medical advice should be sought for a patient who is slow to recover.

Epileptic fits

The epileptic fit is a common cause of loss of consciousness. It is readily distinguished from the simple fainting attack because it is entirely different in character, a convulsive stage preceding the stage of coma. During the convulsive period there are involuntary spasmodic contractions of muscles. The patient may be a known epileptic with a history of previous similar attacks.

There are certain stages of an epileptic seizure. The first of these may be known only to the patient. Its exact nature is peculiar to the patient and it is described as an 'aura'– it takes the form of a sensory disturbance of some type (for example a feeling of dizziness, a visual phenomenon such as flashes of light before the eyes, or a general sensation of unease. It is a warning to the patient that a fit is about to occur.

The warning is followed rapidly by the next stage of the fit. The patient usually cries out and then becomes unconscious. In this stage, which lasts for about half a minute, the patient is rigid and cyanosed, respiration having ceased, and the eyes are turned upwards.

The stage following is the convulsive one in which violent spasmodic movements of the limbs and body occur. Foam appears at the patient's mouth, and there may be incontinence of urine or faeces. This stage lasts for about a minute, and is succeeded by a stage of coma and often sleep.

The first aid treatment of any convulsive type of fit is directed to preventing injury to the patient if and when they become unconscious and during the convulsive stage. The patient with an epileptic seizure will probably have fallen to the ground by the time it is realized that they are having a fit, unless of course they were already lying down. If the patient has not fallen into a position of danger, they need not be moved and tight clothing should be loosened.

When the convulsive stage is reached, the movements of the limbs should not be restrained unless they are likely to result in injury to the patient. The spasms may cause a patient lying on an X-ray table to fall off, and care must be exercised to prevent this happening.

Do not put anything into the patient's mouth and do not try to rouse them from an unconscious state. The convulsive stage of the fit lasts for about a minute and then the muscles relax and the patient remains unconscious. It will take several minutes before a return to consciousness and it may be as long as an hour before the patient is fully recovered.

When the fit is over, the patient should be allowed to rest. The occurrence of the fit should be reported and the patient (even if a known epileptic) should not be allowed to go home unaccompanied.

As well as the major epilepsy which has been described, there is a condition known as minor epilepsy in which the patient has loss of consciousness without the convulsive movements, the unconscious stage being very brief. (The name *grand mal* is sometimes given to major epilepsy, and *petit mal* to the minor variant.)

Asphyxia

Asphyxia is a condition in which the patient lacks oxygen for the body-tissues (*hypoxia*) and it can quickly be fatal if it is not relieved. The state may arise in various ways as enumcratcd below.

(1) The airways and lungs are unable to convey oxygen because they are obstructed internally or externally or because there is fluid in them or because they are compressed (foreign bodies, suffocation, drowning, strangulation, crush injuries to the chest).
(2) The control of respiration through the brain and central nervous system is affected (poisoning, spinal cord injuries, electric shock injuries, cerebral haemorrhage, cerebral thrombosis).
(3) Oxygen is unavailable (gas-filled, smoke-filled rooms and places) or cannot be effectively used by the body (carbon monoxide poisoning, cyanide poisoning).

A patient who is asphyxiating will have obvious difficulty in breathing: the rate and the depth of the respiration increase and it becomes noisy instead of soundless. The patient becomes cyanotic and froth may form around the mouth. The nostrils will be flared and the patient may appear confused and very distressed. This will lead to unconsciousness and, in turn, respiratory arrest.

The first step in aiding a patient in this condition is to remove the cause of the asphyxia if this can be done, and to send for medical assistance. It should be made certain that the airway is clear, and it may be of help to give oxygen by mask. If the patient stops breathing some form of artificial respiration must be started immediately. The method of expired air resuscitation ('mouth-to-mouth breathing') is described in an earlier part of this chapter under the heading Radiological emergencies.

Fractures

In medical terminology the word fracture means a broken bone. There are many types of fracture which can occur, some of them differentiated by special names, usually the name of someone who first described the fracture in relation to certain bones and certain displacements of the broken parts. Examples are Colles' fracture, involving the distal ends of radius and ulna, and Pott's fracture, involving the distal ends of the tibia and fibula. The radiographer will often see such terms on request forms for X-ray examination of injured patients.

However, there are two *general* classifications of fractures which are important. Either the fracture is a *simple* one in which there is no communication between the fracture site and the open air; or it is a *compound* fracture in which there *is* communication between the fracture site and the open air through a skin wound.

Other considerations being equal, a compound fracture is the more serious injury, being liable to infection. No simple fracture should be allowed to become a compound one through careless handling. Any open wound should be covered as soon as possible with a sterile dressing; if this is not available a clean dry dressing must be applied.

Other important general classifications are: complicated fractures (there is an associated injury to an adjacent important organ); comminuted fractures (the bones are fragmented and crushed into several small pieces); greenstick fractures, commonly encountered in children (one edge of a bone is broken and the opposing edge is simply bent).

The signs of a fracture include pain and tenderness at the site of the injury, loss of function, swelling, bruising, obvious deformity of the part. A doctor during examination may discover the unnatural movement between parts of a bone which gives further indication that a fracture has occurred. Some degree of shock may be present.

If an accident occurs in the X-ray department and there is suspicion or certainty that the patient has a fracture, they must be referred for examination, and treatment by a doctor. In the meanwhile the immediate care given must ensure that there is no aggravation of the injury, that no simple fracture is made compound, and that no movement takes place at the fracture site. Such movement can increase the degree of bony displacement which may already have occurred, and can cause the broken ends of bone to damage blood vessels, muscles, and nerves, and may result in bone piercing the skin and producing a compound fracture. In the event of there being doubt as to whether the patient has a fracture, they should be treated as if the injury were a fracture until it is proved otherwise.

These governing principles mean that the injured part must be adequately supported and immobilized when handling and moving the patient, and use must be made of splints and slings where necessary. If the patient has to be lifted the lift must be properly assessed so that the patient can be moved smoothly and without risk. The patient should be reassured and kept warm and comfortable.

Electric shock

An electric shock is the result of an electric current passing through the body. Electricity at a high voltage is dangerous, but it is not the high voltage itself which causes injury, but the current through the body which is produced by the high voltage in certain circumstances. These circumstances may exist when there is failure in protective systems incorporated in electrical apparatus.

Such apparatus is usually made safe to handle by two features.

(1) It is insulated. This means in general that the electrical conductors comprising the circuit are enclosed in non-conducting material, for example the sheathing on electric flex for lamps and fires and on the supply cables of X-ray sets.
(2) Some part of the circuit is earthed. This may be done by connecting it to a metal plate buried in the ground or to a pipe (such as a water main) which goes into the ground. The earth can absorb a vast amount of electric charge, and connection of the apparatus to earth is a measure for the safety of those using it.

There is a tendency for electricity to escape to earth, and where there is failure in the provided safety devices, the path of least resistance may be through the body of someone handling the equipment. So an electric current passes through this person, and the degree of electric shock received depends on the strength of the current. If the body offers a high resistance to the passage of electricity, then the current will be low and the shock will be slight. If the body offers a low resistance to the passage of electricity, then the current will be high and the shock severe. Assuming the resistance of the body to be constant, a higher voltage produces a higher current.

An electric current acts upon the muscles of the body and causes them to contract. In this way the victim of the shock may be unable to breathe because the respiratory muscles are affected, and his heart may stop beating because the heart muscle is involved.

The first thing to do immediately for the victim of an electric shock who is still in contact with the circuit is to switch off the supply at the mains switch, so that the apparatus is no longer 'live'. In the X-ray department it will generally be possible to do this.

If for some reason it is not possible to cut off the supply and the patient has to be pulled away from the apparatus while it is still 'live', unless the rescuer is insulated from the current there will quickly be *two* victims of electric shock. The rescuer should therefore stand upon some insulating material – a cork or rubber mat or a thick blanket. This is particularly important if the floor is wet. A dry wooden floor and a dry floor with a rubber surface both provide reasonable insulation for mains voltage. A dry floor made of polyvinyl tiles provides insulation for voltages below 1000 volts, and therefore gives protection at mains voltage level.

The patient should be pulled away by the clothing and the rescuer's hands should be protected by insulating material, for example rubber or cloth. All articles used for the purpose of insulation must be *dry*. In the X-ray department lead–rubber aprons and gloves may be readily available, and may suggest themselves as suitable material for insulation. Lead–rubber will be adequate for voltages up to 400 volts, but is not reliable protection in the case of high voltage sources. It would be reasonable to use it if the electrical apparatus concerned were operating on the 240 volt mains supply. It should be realized that in the case of a.c. supplies the stated mains voltage is not the highest value reached during the a.c. cycle. The voltage increases to a peak value which is equal to the stated value multiplied by the factor 1.41. In the design of equipment, insulation requirements are based on peak values of voltage.

Once the patient has been rescued from the source of the current, the treatment required will depend upon the injury sustained. The conditions which may be present are:

(1) Cardiac arrest,
(2) Respiratory arrest,
(3) Burns,
(4) Fractures,
(5) Shock.

The rule in all first air procedures is to treat the most serious condition first, and (1) and (2), above, clearly require *immediate* assistance; (3), (4) and (5) are of less urgency.

It is wise to regard electric shock seriously even if the results do not seem to be very severe, and to refer the patient for medical attention.

References

Coady, E. (1994) Artificial ventilation and chest compression. *Nursing Times*, 90 (17) 36–8.

Marsden, A.K., Moffat, C. & Scott, R. (1992) *First Aid Manual*, (page 38), 6th Edn., St John/St Andrew's Ambulance Association & British Red. Cross.

Tortora, G.I. & Anagnostakos, N.P. (1990) *Principles of Anatomy & Physiology*, (page 620), 6th Edn., Harper Collins, London.

Further reading

Dickerson, M. (1988) Anaphylaxis and anaphylactic shock. *Critical Care Nursing Quarterly*, 11 (1), 68–74.

Flanders, A. (1994) A detailed explanation of defibrillation. *Nursing Times*, 90 (18), 37–9.

Maxwell, M. (1983) Everything you need to know about shock. *Nursing Mirror*, March 23, 17–19.

Chapter 18
Medico-legal Aspects of the Radiographer's Work

Reference to the medico–legal aspects of a radiographer's work may induce a sense of panic in the newcomer who feels uncertain of the implications of this alarming phrase. In fact it is necessary to understand in this only certain broad aspects of the radiographer's responsibility towards patients. It is, however, important that these aspects are fully understood, and they may be considered simply under three headings. These are:

(1) Breach of professional confidence;
(2) Negligence;
(3) Procedure in the event of an accident.

Breach of professional confidence

Most people realize that doctors and others in medical work are given knowledge concerning the personal history of those who consult them, and that they must regard such knowledge as strictly confidential. This bond of secrecy applies not only to medical details but to anything which the professional may discover about a patient during consultation and 'treatment.

When a clinician refers a patient to the X-ray department for diagnostic examination, although the patient may never see the radiologist, that patient is in fact being referred for a radiological opinion. This opinion is related to appearances on radiographs or other diagnostic images and is a statement from the radiologist as to the conditions which in his or her belief, are seen to be present; these conditions may be normal or pathological.

In order to come to a well-informed opinion the radiologist must be admitted to the clinician's confidence, and therefore must be told facts about the patient relevant to diagnosis and treatment. Similarly the clinician is admitted to the confidence of the radiographer, who tells the clinician his opinion based on the appearances revealed by the examination which has been made. There is thus an exchange of confidential information, and these matters are properly within the triangle formed by the radiologist, the clinician, and the patient.

Radiographers work closely with the radiologist, and in order that they may perform their duties they too are admitted into this area of confidence. Even the newest student in the department should realize that the work, through reports and case notes, gives access to information about the patient which must always be regarded as confidential. In the United Kingdom radiographers are State Registered, and one of the statutory functions of the Board which registers radiographers concerns itself with standards of professional conduct. It has been specifically stated by the committee concerned with these matters that one of the acts of infamous conduct by a radiographer would be knowingly to 'disclose to any patient, or to any other unauthorized person, the result of any investigations or any other information of a personal or confidential nature gained in the course of practice' of the radiographer's profession (Radiographers Board, 1993).

Strictly there are only two people with whom radiographers may freely discuss a patient and the details of his condition and case history; these two people are the referring clinician and the radiologist to whom the patient has been referred. In practice of course some discussion of patients must fairly and necessarily take place between various other members of the hospital staff; for example between junior radiographers and their seniors, and between radiographers and other nursing staff in whose charge the patients rest. These are legitimate extensions of the triangle of confidence previously mentioned.

The Radiographers Board now recognizes that there may be certain local protocols which allow radiographers to comment on films or images which they have produced. Such protocols normally *do not* extend to student radiographers but allow experienced, qualified radiographers to extend their roles in certain departments under locally agreed circumstances. Such circumstances could include reporting on ultrasound images by trained sonographers or the use of what are known as 'red-dot systems' whereby qualified radiographers indicate that they have observed an anomaly such as a fracture on a radiograph of a casualty patient.

No detail concerning a patient should ever be discussed with another patient or discussed outside the hospital. This applies (as has been said) not only to information on the patient's medical history, but also to anything which may be discovered about a patient in the course of duty. The student radiographer **must** recognize this obligation. This is the 'duty of confidentiality' which civil law places on all health care professionals. This duty extends after the patient's death and professionals can be sued for breaches of confidentiality.

Patients of course ask radiographers questions about examinations which have been made in the department and seek information on what has been revealed. It is quite wrong to escape in the answer that 'they are all right'. Information on the appearance of diagnostic images may only be given to the patient by the radiographer under specific locally agreed schemes of work (see Appendix 1, Clause 4.5). If you, as a student radiographer, are faced with such questioning and are not able to refer the patient to a senior radiographer, the question may be turned aside by some reply such as 'The doctor will see the films and he will be able to tell you', or 'I'm afraid we can't say until the doctor has seen the films all together'. Such answers should be made in as reassuring a manner as possible.

This issue is a little controversial. Some radiographers are uncomfortable with it and others have accused health care professionals of 'hiding behind their white coats' when patients request information. It is important to recognize two things:

(1) The clinician is the best person to discuss a patient's condition with them. Diagnostic radiographers in particular tend to have fairly short periods of contact with individual patients which are certainly not long enough to allow the radiographer to assess how the patient may react to news of their condition. Even a seemingly minor fracture may have serious personal implications for an individual patient. Think, for example, about an elderly patient living alone who may have fractured a metatarsal. This will result in the patient having to wear plaster of paris; this has all sorts of implications for that individual in terms of their ability to cope with everyday life during the period of healing. When seen in this context, the casual giving of such information may be regarded as actual negligence and a failure of our duty of care to the patient, as can be seen in (2) below.

(2) The radiographer needs to be careful not to divulge information about a patient's diagnosis – careful that we do not fail the patient who is merely seeking the opportunity to talk about the worries and fears they may have about their condition. It is critical that we do not deny patients this or we become guilty of the mentality which makes us start conversations with such statements as, 'I'm only the radiographer...'. As health care professionals we also have a duty to care for the patient's psychological well-being. If the radiographer is concerned about inadvertently divulging information, but recognizes the patient's need to talk about their fears/anxieties, then it is the duty of that radiographer to ensure that the patient is referred on to another health care professional who will have the skills to enable the patient to talk through these issues. This person may be a radiologist, the patient's clinician or another professional such as the ward sister.

Negligence

Negligence in this context is simply a failure in care, a failure that arises by doing something (or failing to do something) that no reasonable person would do (or fail to do). In certain cases negligence becomes actionable in civil law. Negligence is actionable when there is a duty to take care, cast by law on someone or some people, and there is a failure in that duty resulting in injury to another person or to others. In all our activities we have a duty to take care to avoid acts or omissions reasonably foreseeable as likely to injure others; this duty is based upon probabilities, not upon bare possibilities.

The Health and Safety at Work Act 1974 places a duty of care upon us in looking out for both our own safety and the safety of others, for example.

The degree of care required from us in law differs in different situations. The factors influencing this degree of care include (1) the risk involved, (2) the known characteristics of persons exposed to risk, and (3) the necessity. Those who do things intrinsically dangerous must exercise a higher degree of care, and certain groups of people will demand more care than others. The standard of care required in law is not the highest possible to which one can conceivably be expected to conform, nor is it the lowest standard of which one is actually capable. It is between these two extremes – the standard of 'the reasonable man'.

Radiographers must recognize that in their work they are certainly placed in the category of those who of necessity submit others to procedures which are intrinsically dangerous. Furthermore, the people who suffer these procedures have known characteristics which demand a higher degree of care. Children, old people, sick people of any age coming to the X-ray department as frightened strangers (for so they must be regarded) certainly need special care. The test to be applied is the foreseeability of injury to others, and any reasonable person would see that hospital patients need a special degree of care – even in as simple a matter as getting on or off an X-ray table – if foreseeable injury is to be prevented (see Fig. 18.1).

We must therefore give attention to detail in all aspects of our care for patients; not only in the technical procedures and use of our equipment, but in matters such as helping the patient in and out of the examination room and as they go about the department. A radiographer who leaves even the most able patient alone to get down from the X-ray table after the simplest examination is as guilty of negligence as the one who fails to check the contrast agent injected for an intravenous urogram; the first situation has just as much possibility of foreseeable injury as the second. We are failing in our legal duties (quite apart from our humane responsibilities) if we do not keep this always in mind.

In using equipment, radiographers have the duty of checking the controls before a diagnostic exposure is made or a treatment is given. In a judgement made in a specific case, the law placed this responsibility firmly on the shoulders of the radiographer, and it was said that all controls must be checked, including those customarily kept on one setting and not usually varied. Although in this particular case reference was made to the controls,

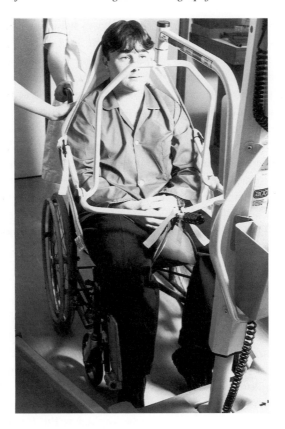

Fig. 18.1 Ensuring patient safety.

the term should be interpreted as referring to *all* aspects of the equipment. This includes simple mechanical features such as the security and working order of such attachments as steps, hand-grips, shoulder-pieces, cones, and diaphragms. Protestations from a patient as to their lack of security on the X-ray table should never be ignored, and attention should be paid even to such non-technical considerations as the risk from a highly polished floor in the examination room.

Another aspect of negligence is failure to read properly requests for X-ray examinations. We all know the importance of this but in practice it may require an effort of conscientiousness from a busy radiographer seeing with dismay some illegible handwriting; but the effort must be made. If, for example, there is a request to 'x-ray the pelvis please' and we fail to elucidate the last erratic line which says 'Stone in the lower end of the ureter', we can take a useless radiograph and submit the patient to a dose of radiation which is not necessary. This is failure in care where there is a duty of care – in one word, negligence.

Equally there is a failure in the duty of care if we do not properly ensure that we have the correct patient at the beginning of an examination. Each patient must be asked to say their name in full, not merely asked if they are the patient whose name appears on the card. Subsequent to this the patient should be asked to give you their home address so that there is a second check that this is indeed the patient to whom the request card refers. The radiographers may then be asked to sign the card to indicate that they have carried out this procedure. Any temptation to short-cut this procedure must be resisted – remember: subjecting a patient to an unnecessary dose of radiation constitutes negligence and as such is a very serious matter.

Negligence occurs, too, when a radiographer uses X-ray equipment without complete precautions to reduce to its necessary minimum the radiation dose received by the patient. There is certainly a duty of care in the use of radiation which our special knowledge fits us to meet and we must not fail to meet it.

Responsibility for negligence

We are each of us personally responsible for any negligence of which we are guilty. In law an employer may also be vicariously responsible for the negligent acts or omissions of those he employs (called in this context his servants) when these acts occur within the scope of their work. This vicarious responsibility does not make the servants of the employer immune.

Radiographers in the National Health Service in the United Kingdom are considered in law as the servants of the hospital trust employing them. This means that if a radiographer is negligent, and a patient suffers injury as a result, in most cases the responsibility will be assumed by the employing hospital authority. If legal proceedings follow and damages are awarded to the injured patient, the hospital authority is liable for payment of these damages. There is, however, nothing in law to prevent the hospital authority from seeking to recover the damages from its servants. Such cases have occurred, a judgement being given in a specific case (not involving a radiographer) for an employing authority to secure a contribution of 100% of the damages from its servant. It is possible too for the name of a radiographer to be joined with a hospital authority in a legal action, the radiographer being liable with the employing authority for damages claimed. This has occurred in a particular case.

These facts may sound alarming, but it is possible for radiographers to insure themselves against this type of risk; membership of certain professional bodies carries such insurance. The risk may not be very great, but radiographers considering the medico-legal aspects of their work should fully appreciate that it exists.

Membership of a profession such as radiography requires certain standards of professional conduct. The Society of Radiographers in the United Kingdom publishes a code of professional conduct to which its members are expected to work. The Code is included as an Appendix of this book. Professional bodies in other countries such as the United States have similar codes of conduct.

Procedure in the event of an accident

It is obvious that even in the best X-ray department staffed by the least negligent radiographers accidents can and will happen, both to patients and to personnel. The procedures in such cases are in three sections.

(1) Care for the victim.
(2) Reporting the accident.
(3) Recording the accident.

Care for the victim is advisedly placed first, and is to be given immediately, however slight the injury may seem to be. Detailed procedures in first aid and treatment clearly will be determined by what has happened, and need not be discussed here. Even if the accident seems trivial and the injury slight, it is wise to seek medical advice as part of the care of the victim.

Reporting and recording the accident may here be considered together. They are both extremely important. It must be done with complete honesty and frankness if the reports and the records are to be of any value at all.

In the United Kingdom, since 1981 there have been certain legal requirements with which health authorities and hospitals must comply in regard to accidents and dangerous occurrences which happen on their premises. These requirements are encompassed within the Reporting of Injuries, Disease & Dangerous Occurrences Regulations (1985), known as RIDDOR. The RIDDOR regulations require that information about an accident or dangerous incident (see categories below) be passed to the Health & Safety Executive, who will then institute their own investigation, monitoring and enforcing safety procedures for the protection of employees and the general public. Failure to follow these rules constitutes a breach of the law. Many other countries have similar statutes and procedures.

In the United Kingdom there are four main categories of incidents for which these procedures have been stipulated. These are as follows.

(1) Dangerous occurrences. This is a term which embraces a number of clearly defined events such as the following: the collapse or overturning of a crane or a hoist (the collapse of a ceiling mounted X-ray tubestand would be an example within a radiographic department); bursting of a

boiler; fire or explosion; collapse of a building or a part of it; uncontrolled escapes of dangerous agents; occupational exposure to pathogens which results in acute ill-health.

(2) Fatal accidents. These accidents are by definition those in which human life is lost.

(3) Major injury accidents. Major injuries are defined in the regulations and include fractures of the spine, the skull, the pelvis, arms and legs; amputations of limbs; loss of sight of an eye; other injuries which involve admission to hospital for longer than 24 hours.

(4) Other accidents.

The first steps of the procedures which are stipulated by the regulations indicate a reporting sequence which, once initiated, leads to records being made through the completion of the required report form. The sequence is as follows.

(1) Accident or dangerous occurrence happens;

(2) Report at once to the most senior person available in the department at the time;

(3) This senior person investigates the incident and, at once,

(4) Completes Part 1 of the Report Form;

(5) A doctor giving treatment immediately then completes Part 2 of the Report Form;

(6) Report is made to the head of the department who checks the Report form, and

(7) completes Part 3 of the Report Form, retaining a copy;

(8) A designated hospital administrator receives the report from the head of the department within 5 days of the incident;

(9) Hospital administrators must maintain a register of all these accidents and dangerous occurrences, the registers being annually reviewed.

The essential information embodied in the Report Form provides written answers to questions which arise, such as the following.

(1) What happened?

(2) When and where did it happen?

(3) Who and what were involved?

(4) Who was present?

(5) What was the outcome?

(6) What actions were taken?

The usefulness of the written account is twofold. Firstly, if any legal action arises out of the matter there will be available a permanent record of what the situation was at the time and what measures were taken. Secondly a clear account of the circumstances of the accident may serve to show how it has occurred. This may focus attention on some feature of the department – its equipment, its organization, its conditions, its practices, its staff situation – which made the accident more likely to occur and should be improved for safety. Through this it may be possible to stop the event repeating itself at a later date.

When an accident happens, particularly if it is a very alarming and serious accident, it is not always easy to report correctly afterwards exactly what has occurred. As trained people, radiographers must try to meet these situations as coolly as they can, and to retain unimpaired their faculties of judgement and observation.

The importance of records

From this particular case of recording an accident, it may be useful to proceed further to consider the importance of all records kept in hospital and in the X-ray department. The diagnostic radiograph is itself a record, a record of certain conditions existing within the body of a particular patient at the time the examination was made. The radiographic record (if it is to have value) must be completely identified as to the patient, the date, and the circumstances – for example its place in an intravenous urogram series or other sequence. It must also be capable of being found if needed. The record systems and arrangements for film-marking and filing used in X-ray departments are directed towards these ends.

Patients' records in hospital are intended partly for the transmission of information. This is done more clearly and with more saving in time and effort if the transmission is by written and not simply by spoken words. Another purpose of these records is the provision of a permanent account so that for diagnosis and treatment comparisons may be made between the patient's condition at different times. These permanent written records are independent of such factors as change in staff and in hospitals – the patient may be seeing another doctor in another place at a different time – and the fallibility of human memory.

Beyond the individual patient there is a much wider field of use for many types of hospital record and hospital statistics. Without them it would be impossible for medical science to advance, for financial assessments to be made, for services to be planned and developed to meet demands which are predictable by studying the records of previous activity.

In the X-ray department efficient (or even merely adequate) administration requires the keeping of records other than simple documentation of patients. For example, maintenance and renewal of equipment, supplies of films, chemicals, and drugs, movements of staff, holiday dates, personnel monitoring as part of radiation protection, collections of radiographs showing various abnormal and normal conditions – all these respects of departmental work require detailed record systems of their own which are independent of changes in time and in staff.

While the keeping of records may often seem trivial, tedious, and consuming of time and energy upon which many claims are made, it must be appreciated that attention given to the task is by no means wasted. Records are of value and significance not only in particular instances, but generally in the provision of a competent service to patients, and, as has been seen this is primarily the purpose of a hospital's existence and useful function.

Increasingly, the keeping of such records is by means of a computerized administration system which may encompass not only the management of all patient records but also the monitoring of equipment and film supplies and other administrative details as mentioned above. The use of such systems may speed up the throughput of departments and improve their administration, but they create their own demands (Marsh, 1989; Crowe, 1993).

References

Crowe, H. (1993) An evaluation of data input errors by radiographers using a patient administration system. *Radiography Today*, 59 (676), 19–22.

Marsh, A.J. (1989) Developing a radiology computer system. *Radiography Today*, 55 (622), 20–22.

Radiographers Board (1993) *Statement On Infamous Conduct*. Council For Professions Supplementary to Medicine.

Further reading including relevant legislation

Control of Substance Hazardous to Health (COSHH) Regulations 1988

Health & Safety at Work Act 1974

Reporting of Injuries, Disease & Dangerous Occurrences Regulations (RIDDOR) 1985.

Ryan, A., in Tortorici, M. (1992) *Concepts in Medical Radiographic Imaging*, (Chapter 17, Computerizing Administrative Tasks), WB Saunders Co, Philadelphia.

Chapter 19
The Patient and the Radiation Hazard

Even before their acceptance as candidates for training, most student radiographers are aware that the radiations with which they will work have the capacity to harm, and that excessive exposure to them will damage human tissue. Indeed this aspect of the work is one not only familiar to those occupationally in contact with ionizing radiations, but also widely known to the public at large. In many instances patients are sufficiently aware of the harmful potential of X-radiation to become anxious and alarmed if what appears a large number of radiographs have to be taken.

The nature of the risk

In diagnostic X-ray examinations we are not concerned with doses of radiation within the 'excessive' category. To mention, as one instance, a radiation effect of which the public generally is cognizant, we are unlikely to produce sterility in a patient as a result of any diagnostic radiological procedure. However, in recent years the attention of research workers has been directed towards hazards which may be produced by low levels of irradiation and which subjects undergoing diagnostic radiography may well incur.

These risks are dual in nature. The first is *genetic*, or hereditary, that is, it refers to the possibility of undesirable effects upon a future generation, and it arises because of the ability of X-rays – and other ionizing radiations – to bring about certain changes, known as *mutations*, in reproductive cells. Such slight alteration in the reproductive cells of each of a large number of subjects could lead to the existence of inherited defects in their descendants, not immediately apparent in their children but becoming manifest in the individuals of a far later generation.

In any population there is a certain mutation rate which is said to occur naturally. It is thought at present that perceptible genetic damage would occur if there were irradiation of the whole populace sufficient to raise the natural mutation rate to twice its present level.

Everyone receives naturally a small dose of radiation from the environment, due to cosmic rays, radioactive materials in the earth's crust and traces of radioactivity within the body which are present as the result of small amounts of radioactive substances in water, food and the atmosphere. This is an inevitable background dose to which we are all subject. In addition, many people receive radiation from the man-made sources. Reports show that the largest man-made contribution to the genetic hazard comes from medical radiology (Sumner, 1987).

Over the world as a whole this contribution is 20% of the level received from natural resources; but in those countries where extensive medical services are available the figure approaches 50%. This is a degree of population exposure to radiation which none of us may disregard and which requires the unremitting attention of every radiographer, no matter how trivial may seem the particular procedure at the moment concerned. Results which are neither tangible nor likely to become evident within a lifetime are prone to lack significance for us. It is important that we each are actively aware of the reality of this obligation towards our patients, and that we take every step to ensure that the radiation dose received in the course of *any* diagnostic X-ray examination is never higher than it need be.

The second type of hazard to which research workers have given recent attention is that termed *somatic*. This refers to delayed effects which may be seen in an irradiated subject after some varying period of time, perhaps many years, following exposure. At the present time it is not well understood whether these delayed effects are ever caused by low levels of exposure and clearly it is difficult to obtain clear-cut evidence on such a point. In the absence of proof it is necessary – because we cannot safely do otherwise – to assume that low levels of irradiation *can* product somatic damage.

The effects of exposure to radiation are sometimes classified in *stochastic* and *non-stochastic categories*. A stochastic effect is one for which the probability of occurrence is seen as a function of dose: there is no threshold level of dose, below which the effect is without clinical significance; and thus there is no level of irradiation which may be called 'safe'. The non-stochastic effects of ionizing radiation are those of which the severity varies in proportion to the dose and for which a threshold of risk may be identified.

Genetic effects, and most somatic effects associated with the dose levels of medical radiodiagnosis, are stochastic. The goals of radiation protection have been described as:

(1) The prevention of detrimental non-stochastic effects;
(2) To hold the probability of stochastic effects within an acceptable level.

Naturally the problem with (2) above lies in the question: what is an acceptable level of risk? (Milner, 1989.)

There can be no answer to this in universal terms, since the acceptability of the risk is in a balance with the potential benefit to the patient concerned; and benefit cannot be quantified. Consequently the judgement to be made is qualitative. Anyone who initiates an X-ray examination should first have asked of himself the question: will this procedure result in a benefit to the patient which outweighs the radiation risk? Medical diagnostic radiology has become the significant specialty that it is because doctors have found that the answer to this question usually is 'Yes'.

However, it is in the hands of radiographers that the faithful practice of radiation protection indisputably lies: in nearly every circumstance, the finger on the exposure switch is a radiographer's. All exposures should be kept as low as reasonably achievable. This is known as the ALARA (as low as reasonably achievable) principle (Milner, 1989).

Measures taken to minimize the genetic hazard from medical radiology, in general will minimize also the somatic risk. In what follows consideration is given mainly to the possibility of damage of the genetic kind.

It must be recognized that our awareness of the genetic risk and our concern to avoid unnecessary irradiation of those of child-bearing age should not sanction the acceptance of an incomplete examination. However, it is now recognized that there is a need to place some restraint on the numbers and extent of some requests for radiological investigations. The new guidelines published by the Royal College of Radiologists (RCR Working Party, 1993) highlight the fact that at present a significant number of requests do nothing to contribute to patient management and give reasons for this which include doing the wrong study for the clinical indications and failing to explain fully the purpose of the examination. The guidelines are discussed in the context of minimizing radiation dose and other factors such as the medico-legal position. The resource implications of ineffective examinations are also pointed out. It is also made clear that these are guidelines, not regulations, but that clinicians do have to have good reasons for choosing to ignore them.

Radiography of the pregnant

X-ray examination of a woman who is known or thought to be pregnant creates a particular problem in radiation protection because the radiation risk has special aspects. It is known that the maturing human embryo is potentially sensitive to ionizing radiations. The possibility exists of fetal malformations being produced as the result of a radiation dose delivered to the mother for the purpose of a diagnostic radiological examination. This is damage in the *somatic* category. It may be presumed that the *genetic* risk to a fetus is not greater than for other irradiated subjects.

It is thought that there is a period which is critical during embryonic development. It may be that there are a number of critical periods in the maturing of an embryo, embryonic organ or tissue, but knowledge of these matters is not yet complete. We do not know exactly when this critical period is: all we can say at present is that a fetus is at greater risk from irradiation early in intra-uterine life than when it is almost or fully mature. Ionizing radiations are known to alter chromosomes. As these control fetal development there may be a direct connection between such irradiation and chromosomal abnormalities resulting in a malformed child.

There are some grounds for believing that irradiation of the fetus *in utero* carries another risk. It has been suggested that leukaemia and other malignant diseases occur a little more often in children whose mothers have been subjected to diagnostic radiological examinations during the pregnancy.

For these reasons, X-ray investigations of pregnant women should be carefully controlled along the following lines.

(1) Unless the condition is one requiring immediate attention such patients should not have X-ray examinations of the abdomen, lumbar spine or pelvic regions, particularly procedures involving serial films or fluoroscopy: for example, tomography, intravenous urography, myelography and barium studies (RCR Working Party, 1993).

(2) When a pregnant woman is referred to the X-ray department for obstetric reasons, repeat films should be avoided if possible and there is thus a special charge on the radiographer to obtain satisfactory radiographs in the first instance.

(3) When the examination is not directly of the uterus or pelvis, for example during radiography of the lung fields or teeth, the radiographer has an unavoidable moral responsibility to protect the fetus as far as possible from both direct and secondary radiation by providing a suitable lead–rubber apron for the patient.

(4) If the patient is known to be pregnant, failure to inform the department of diagnostic radiology of this fact may be taken as negligence on the part of the referring clinician (RCR Working Party, 1993).

During the first month of pregnancy there is a very small risk – not considered to need special measures – of a fertilized ovum failing to implant in the uterus; during the second month, detriment caused by irradiation is taken to refer to the malformation of specific organs; during the third and fourth months of the pregnancy, defective development of the forebrain may lead to lowered intelligence or overt mental retardation in a child.

In 1964 the International Commission on Radiological Protection published (ICRP – 6) its first recommendation about radiation protection of the fetus. This report states that the 10-day interval following the onset of a menstrual period 'is the only time when it is virtually certain that women of such age (reproductive age) are not pregnant'. Later than this date in the cycle, ovulation should normally have occurred and the woman may be carrying a fertilized ovum, though as yet unaware that she is pregnant.

As a consequence of these facts, the Commission then recommended that, in women of reproductive age, non-urgent X-ray examinations entailing irradiation of the lower abdomen and pelvis should be made only during the 10-day interval in the monthly cycle when pregnancy was improbable. In a later publication (ICRP – 9), the term *women of reproductive age* became more realistically *women of reproductive capacity*, but both publications have been widely misinterpreted and restrictively applied as a *ten-day rule*, a term which ICRP itself has never used.

Misunderstanding of the 'rule' arose because practitioners generally failed to appreciate the Commission's definition of a non-essential examination and postponed the investigation of many patients' conditions unless these were of *immediate* medical urgency. The Commission's recommendation in ICRP – 6 actually stated, however, that the examinations which should be delayed were those which – without harm to the patient – might wait until the end of a pregnancy; later publications of the Commission (including ICRP – 9) even specifically remarked that the examinations which it was appropriate to delay were very few. These conclusions were reiterated in joint guidelines (COR/RCR, 1986) which give advice on the diagnostic exposure of women who 'are, or who may be, pregnant'. The guidelines require the introduction of an agreed procedure for each department for diagnostic examinations of women falling within this category. This requires the examining radiographer to ask any woman of reproductive capacity (in cases where the uterus is likely to be in, or near, the primary beam) whether there is any possibility that she might be pregnant. If she gives an affirmative answer then the case is referred back, via the radiologist, to the referring clinician to determine whether the examination should proceed. (This has become known colloquially as the '28 – day rule').

The radiography of children

Children are presumed to have more years of life ahead of them than adults. Because of this longer life expectancy, they may be considered to have an enlarged potential for the manifestation of radiation damage; this gives a special concern to the radiation protection of children during diagnostic X-ray investigations, notwithstanding that the radiation dose used for the examination of a child is likely to be smaller than if the patient were an adult.

The most effective provision of radiation protection to any patient consists in not X-raying him: it is particularly important in the case of a child that no one should make an X-ray examination which is questionable in value. The primary decision 'to X-ray' or 'not to X-ray' is not taken by radiographers: their responsibility – once the decision has been made and the patient comes to the X-ray department – comprises the production of clear radiographs; that is, the avoidance of images of such dubious quality that a doctor's clinical uncertainty is exchanged for a radiological doubt.

Overall, the commonest reason to repeat a radiograph is because the density and contrast of the image are unacceptable in some respect; that is, exposure selection was incorrectly made.

Unless the radiographer is experienced in paediatrics and perhaps is working in a department where many patients – or even all patients – are children, this common ground of error is trapped with the pitfalls of transposing radiographic exposure factors from adults to children of various ages and sizes. Particular care must be used if a repeat examination is to be avoided.

Detail sharpness in a radiographic image may be unsatisfactory because the subject has moved during the exposure. Since children mainly are restless creatures – and some too young to take instruction – the elimination of motional unsharpness from radiographs becomes a significant concern of paediatric radiographers. Three approaches to the problem commonly are made.

(1) **The selection of short exposure intervals.** The importance of these must override some deterioration in radiographic geometry if – in the interests of avoiding an overload of the X-ray tube – it becomes necessary to use a larger focal spot. Generators of low output, since they limit exposure selection unduly, are undesirable for paediatric radiography.

(2) **The use of accessory equipment and manoeuvres physically to restrain a patient.** Mechanical immobilization in a fixed position has its greater success with babies and young infants; it should not – indeed cannot effectively – be employed to 'win the battle' against a frightened toddler.

(3) **The perpetual avoidance of a 'battle situation' by the radiographer in charge of the examination**; in whom preferably some understanding of children has been cultivated and whose training has acknowledged that the reactions of children and adults are different (Gyll & Blake, 1986).

It is not a function of the present text to analyse these approaches any further: but it is understandable that cases are often made for equipping certain radiodiagnostic rooms particularly for the examination of children; and for enlisting specifically experienced radiographers whenever possible. Undeniably such planning has a part to play in the radiation protection of the young.

Significant examinations

Genetic damage results from irradiation of the reproductive cells and consequently as a rule the most important (though not the only) dose to consider in diagnostic radiography is that received by the gonads of the subject. Those examinations which involve inclusion within the primary beam of the testes in the male and the ovaries in the female are clearly the worst offenders.

Also to be considered is the dose to the gonads from scattered radiation, when the site of examination in fact may be remote from the reproductive organs: for example, during radiography of the chest or teeth. The significance of the patient's position in X-raying the extremities should not be overlooked. For instance, the gonads of a male patient, seated on the X-ray table for radiography of his foot, may be irradiated, owing to the direction towards him of the tilted X-ray tube.

Much time has been given to the assessment of the mean gonad dose incurred during a wide variety of diagnostic X-ray examinations made under different conditions. It has been established:

(1) That when the pelvis is directly irradiated, the gonad dose received by females is greater than that received by males;

(2) That when the dose received by the reproductive organs is due to scattered radiation (as distinct from inclusion of the gonads within the primary beam) then the quantity received by males is greater than that received by females.

Consequently it follows that the radiation risk from any particular X-ray examination is not the same for all patients, but may be greater or less depending upon the sex and size of the subject. For example, during radiography of the lumbar spine, renal tract, gall bladder or abdomen, the female reproductive organs are likely to lie within the primary beam. In examinations of the hip, the male organs most probably will be directly irradiated. Again, the greater gonad dose which may be received in their course makes X-ray examinations of the extremities more significant for males than for females.

Protective measures

The assessment of the dose received by the patient during diagnostic X-ray procedures, and methods by which it may effectively be reduced are complicated matters to which physicists have given serious attention and which no doubt are not properly within the scope of this book. It is, however, easily recognized that to implement such recommendations as may emerge from this work is the hour-to-hour responsibility of the radiographer – whether the most senior member of the department or its newest comer; it is a responsibility which is always with us and of which we should remain constantly aware.

In addition we have a responsibility to others than the patient. We should make use of the protective measures available for ourselves, our colleagues and anyone else who may be immediately concerned with a patient undergoing a diagnostic X-ray examination.

A full consideration of these problems must include a number of aspects which may not be within the immediate control of the radiographer who conducts the examination. These include the output characteristics of a particular X-ray set, the filtration of the primary beam, and the possibility of some leakage of radiation occurring from the tube housing. (This is referred to as 'leakage radiation'). These are nevertheless a few simple measures the observation of which, whenever possible, reduces materially the dose received by the patient.

(1) The use of the fastest imaging system which is consistent with the production of adequate radiographic detail.
(2) The use of gonad shields or similar lead protection when such shielding does not obscure areas of diagnostic importance on the radiograph.
(3) Proper limitation of the area covered by the X-ray beam (Fig. 19.1).
(4) Appropriate use of posteroanterior projections, particularly of the skull: the eyes incur a smaller dose from an occipitofrontal than from a fronto-occipital projection.
(5) The use – when available and appropriate – of a 'freeze and recall' facility during television fluoroscopy.

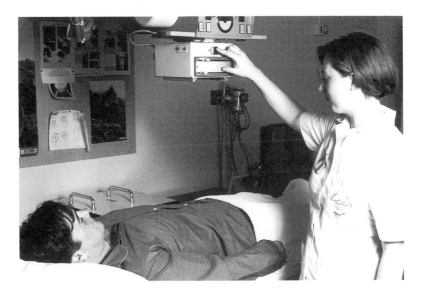

Fig. 19.1 Proper limitation of the area covered by the X-ray beam.

Aprons and gloves

Student radiographers should not be long in X-ray departments before lead-rubber gloves and aprons become familiar items to them. Gloves are to be worn whenever hands – other than those of the patient – must be placed within the area of the primary beam. Like the gloves, the purpose of the aprons is to protect from radiation and they should be worn whenever there is the possibility of unavoidable exposure to secondary radiation. Their use is obligatory in the following situations:

(1) Whenever departmental, nursing, medical or other staff must stand close to a patient whilst an X-ray exposure – radiographic or fluoroscopic – is made;
(2) Whenever a relative, friend, or other member of the public, such as an ambulance officer or a police officer, is required to support a patient during an X-ray examination. If it is feasible, gloves as well as an apron should be worn.

Radiographers should condition themselves not only to putting on their own aprons but to handing an apron to anyone else in the vicinity in the X-ray room, or at the bedside in the ward, or in the casualty room, who may be without one. While members of the X-ray department's staff usually will request or obtain a lead-rubber apron if the occasion requires one, others may not so readily make themselves heard. Outsiders do not fully recognize the risk and hospital staff – especially perhaps junior nursing members – may be reluctant to appear frightened or to give the impression that they are 'making a fuss' unnecessarily. We – who do understand the potential radiation hazard – have a moral duty to see that others are reasonably protected as well as ourselves.

Lead-rubber aprons come in a variety of styles and both they and the gloves should have certain minimum lead equivalents depending upon the kilovoltages generating the X-rays to which they will be exposed. In many countries (including the United Kingdom) certain recommendations are published relating to protection from ionizing radiations and these include among other matters a statement of appropriate lead equivalents for aprons and gloves; for instance, a minimum lead equivalent of 0.25 mm for X-rays generated at voltages up to 150 KV.

Readers of this book should study approved codes relating to the use of ionizing radiation in diagnostic radiology and must be familiar with relevant regulations and the local rules of their own institutes.

Manufacturers supply aprons in many styles and sizes; of lead equivalents ranging from 0.15 mm to 0.5 mm; and of weights varying from 1.1 kilograms ($2\frac{1}{2}$ lb) to 9.3 kilograms (21 lb). Although loosely called aprons, much of this protective clothing is better described as a coatee or jerkin, since it is double-sided and covers the back as well as the front of the wearer; sometimes, in order to make the garment lighter, the lead equivalent of the back may be lower than the front.

The substance used varies in different examples of apron. It may be lead-loaded rubber covered with cloth, or a suitable base impregnated with lead salts and faced with nylon or plastic materials. Plastics – as they are impervious to fluids – have the advantage of being easy to keep clean. Flexibility of the material and general tailoring of the apron are important factors to the comfort of the wearer, since none is light in weight as we usually understand the term and sometimes these aprons are worn for periods of hours.

Care of aprons and gloves

Protective aprons and gloves should be kept clean, stains from contrast agents being those most likely to afflict them. They also should be inspected regularly for evidence of wear, if deteriorated levels of radiation protection are to be avoided.

In X-ray departments in the United Kingdom, an experienced radiographer is usually given special responsibility for radiation safety and should check the condition of gloves and aprons at prescribed intervals. A fluoroscopic inspection will show whether the protection is intact or not, together with the extent of any defect present. In the latter event, the site of the breech – usually a crack of varying length – should be marked on the apron; and a decision must be made regarding future use or replacement of the garment.

Lead aprons are susceptible to damage by creases and folds. They should not be left hanging partially over the edge of a chair-seat or other article of furniture or lying doubled on a shelf. The coatee or two-sided type of apron can be put on a coat hanger but the ordinary variety of hanger is not strong enough for the load: a special hanger can easily be obtained from one apron manufacturer at least. An alternative method of storage is to drape the aprons over a wall-mounted rail, in the way that towels are kept in a bathroom.

The use of gonad shields

Where it is practicable direct shielding of the gonads with a lead sheet is clearly an efficient means of reducing radiation dosage. (Lead-rubber should not be used without a previous check to ensure that it will attenuate the primary beam to a sufficiently low level.) In most abdominal X-ray examinations, if the subject is a male, the scrotum may be shielded without likelihood of obscuring features of diagnostic significance. However, if the patient is a woman there are relatively few examinations involving irradiation of the pelvis and abdomen in which shielding of the ovaries would not be detrimental to the radiograph. In these circumstances it is necessary to rely on other methods of protection.

In the case of a child, gonad shielding may be inadvisable in practice, though theoretically possible. For example, in X-ray examinations made to detect the presence of congenital dislocations of the hip, the area of diagnostic importance is adjacent radiographically to both the testis and the ovary but sufficiently removed from them to permit their shielding – provided such protection can be accurately placed.

This will be recognized as a simple statement which covers sundry difficulties, the major one being that even if correctly placed in the first instance the appropriate lead shield is scarcely likely to remain at its post, when the subject is an active child expressing uninhibited disapproval of the entire procedure. The attempt to use such protection may well entail – through repeat radiographs – a higher dose to the patient than would have been the case had a gonad shield not been used in the first instance.

In some cases it would be desirable to protect the gonads for subsequent examinations, though not for the initial survey. This is true, for example, of accident cases involving the possibility of fractures of the pelvis. Clinical indications may suggest a particular site of bone involvement, but it is unwise to take radiographs only of a strictly localized area. In this type of case the exploratory examination should be made reasonably extensive. Later radiographs of a proven lesion are a different matter and here only the immediate area should be included, unless there are definite indications to the contrary.

There are in common use a number of devices which will protect the gonads from radiation. These most usually take the form of a lead strip, sometimes mounted on a T-shaped or triangular perspex base, which is placed on the patient in an appropriate position over the thighs or lower abdomen. A variant of this is essentially a mask placed at the X-ray beam's exit port from the tube-head (Fig. 19.2); this must operate in conjunction with a light-beam collimator or diaphragm which visually delineates on the subject the area covered by the protector.

Apron protection for the patient

An earlier section of this chapter (see Aprons and Gloves) described the wearing of aprons manufactured from flexible lead-impregnated materials, as a means to reduce the dose received by departmental and other personnel associated with the care of patients during X-ray examinations. In some circumstances a similar apron may be advisable for the patient. The following are appropriate:

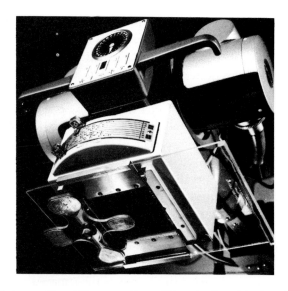

Fig. 19.2 The Leicester Gonad Protector. Four differently shaped lead masks (2 male, 2 female) are incorporated in a rotatable perspex disc. The radiation shielding corresponds to the shadow the lead mask casts when the light beam is in operation. *(Reproduced by courtesy of Picker International Ltd.)*

(1) An apron which can be worn by a patient seated in a chair for the purposes of dental radiography and provides cover for the front of the body from the level of the neck to that of the knees. Such an apron may include a thyroid protector.

(2) A waist apron which can be secured round the patient or suspended during chest radiography. This is particularly recommended when the subject is pregnant but ideally should be used for any individual of child-bearing capacity.

Limitation of the irradiated area

Careful confinement of the radiation field to the area which is diagnostically significant is a valuable contribution to radiation safety which is in the hands of every practising radiographer; it should receive punctilious attention. Thoughtless procedure may easily become established when there is a failure of technical skill.

At the present time most major X-ray equipment is fitted with a beam collimator or diaphragm providing visual evidence of the field size covered by the beam at any anode-film distance. It is important that the radiographer should make intelligent use of this and should by inspection limit the beam to a minimum in every case. If the last use of the unit was made for the same type of radiograph, it is potentially dangerous to assume that the previous setting of the diaphragm will serve again; the new patient may well be smaller than their predecessor (Carter, 1994).

A cassette sensor may be associated with some X-ray tube/bucky combinations; this device means that when a cassette is placed in the bucky tray automatic collimation of the beam then occurs, in order to ensure that the irradiated area is never larger than the cassette to be exposed. Manual override of the system usually is available, so that the area of the beam may be made smaller at the discretion of the radiographer; but a radiographer who intends to rely on the automatic control should take care to select for the examination no larger a cassette than is needed.

For chest radiography many departments, in addition to the light beam unit, employ a gonad screen or apron which is suspended at waist level of the patient and will provide protection of the gonads from the primary beam. However, the presence of such a device does not release the radiographer from the ethical obligation to limit the area of the primary beam in order to avoid undue irradiation of the gonads from scatter.

Equipment employed for fluoroscopy whenever possible should incorporate accessory devices designed to give protection to the patient. These are not to be confused with provisions for the safety of the operator, and they include the following.

(1) A fluoroscopic timing switch which indicates the period during which the patient is actually subjected to fluoroscopy. At the end of a preset limit it will open the fluoroscopic circuit, usually to the accompaniment of a warning buzzer or visual signal from a lamp; sometimes both.

(2) A limiting device which, at any anode-screen distance, prevents opening of the fluoroscopic diaphragms to field size beyond the margins of the image receptor. While primarily of value in protecting the operator and assistants, this device – which provides for a constant visual indication of beam size – clearly operates also in favour of the patient (Carter, 1994).

In some cases an X-ray set may properly be subjected to one or even a number of trial exposures. This may occur, for example, in using portable equipment in an unfamiliar environment when it is desirable before taking a radiograph to make sure that the line fuses will carry the projected load. Or, again, a number of milliampere-meter readings may have to be obtained to check the output of an X-ray equipment thought to be faulty in operation.

When tests of this nature are made it is important beforehand to pay attention to the direction in which the X-ray tube may happen to be aimed at the time. It should never be allowed to remain in line with either a patient or indeed any other person in the room. Where an adjustable diaphragm is fitted, this should be fully closed. Alternatively the tube head may be lowered to the surface of the X-ray table, on which is placed a sheet of lead, or the beam may be directed towards an *outer* wall of the room.

These are simple but important points, the observation of which should become automatic by all who handle X-ray equipment. Only by continuous attention to the radiation hazard can we diminish its risks. Only by constant care in our work can we discharge fully our responsibility to ourselves, our patients, and the generations which will follow. Though remote in its repercussion, we cannot say that the genetic risk does not matter. We have a responsibility for it, which belongs collectively to our age and rests in particular upon each of us as individuals.

References

Carter, P. (1994) *Chesney's Equipment for Student Radiographers*, (pages 89–94, 120–123), 4th Edn., Blackwell Science, Oxford.

COR/RCR (1986) *Guidelines for Implementation of ASP8 Exposure to Ionising Radiation of Pregnant Women: Advice on the Diagnostic Exposure of Women who are, or who may be, Pregnant.*

Gyll, C. & Blake, N. (1986) *Paediatric Diagnostic Imaging*, (Chapter 1), Heinemann, London.

Milner, S. (1989) A strategy for reduction of radiation to patients due to diagnostic X-ray exposures. *Radiography Today*, 55 (630), 19–20.

RCR Working Party (1993) *Making the Best Use of a Department of Clinical Radiology*, 2nd Edn., Royal College of Radiologists, London.

Sumner, D. (1987) *Radiation Risks; an Evaluation*, (pages 61–66), Tarragon Press, Glasgow.

Further reading

Ionizing Radiations Regulations 1985 & 1988.

Colleran, C. (1994) PA lumbar spines – a future concept. *Radiography Today*, 60 (681), 17–20.

Wade, P. (1994) Science and practicalities of patient dose measurement procedures. *Radiography Today*, 60 (681), 13–16.

Appendix
A Code of Professional Conduct for Radiographers

(Published 1994 by the College of Radiographers and reprinted by kind permission)

Introduction

This Code of Professional Conduct is issued by the College of Radiographers to give advice and guidance to all practising members and those studying to gain qualification for state registration. The purpose of the code is to promote voluntary standards of professional behaviour. The code is for guidance only and should not be seen as a definitive statement on professional conduct or behaviour. It should be read in conjunction with the Amended Memorandum and New Articles of Association of The Society of Radiographers (June 1990).

The code is divided into four sections: relationships with, and responsibilities to, patients; professional integrity; professional relationships and responsibilities; professional standards. Each section is subdivided into statements of principle followed, as necessary, by notes which assist in interpreting the principle.

The code replaces any previous code in circulation before 1994.

1. Relationships with, and responsibilities to, patients

1.1 *Confidentiality:* **Radiographers must hold in confidence any information obtained through professional attendance on a patient.**

Radiographers may discuss with the patient information obtained as a result of a diagnostic or therapeutic procedure. Normally this will be in accordance with an agreed scheme of work developed within the employing authority.

If there is a legal requirement to divulge information advice should be sought from your line manager and ultimately from your employer before responding. It is likely that your employer will seek legal advice before responding to you.

If, exceptionally, it is judged necessary to divulge information the consent of the patient should normally be obtained.

Refer to:

current NHS Code of Practice which sets out how to respond to the Act on access to personal health information;
Access to Health Records Act 1990;
Data Protection Act 1984;

The Patient's Charter;
The Radiographers Board Statement on Infamous Conduct.

1.2   *Cruelty:* **Radiographers must not engage in, or condone, behaviour which causes unnecessary mental or physical distress to the patient and their relatives.**

Radiographers must have regard to the physical and psychological needs of patients and their relatives and the effects on them of the hospital environment.

Any examination or treatment likely to cause pain or distress must be explained to the patient or guardian before being undertaken and consent given. Patients should not be left in pain or distress after the examination or treatment, but where this is unavoidable for a short time steps must be taken to provide the appropriate support.

1.3   *Respecting Patients' Rights:* Radiographers have a responsibility to promote and protect the dignity, privacy, autonomy and safety of all patients with whom they come into contact.

Radiographers should have regard to the customs, values, and spiritual beliefs of patients.

Radiographers should at all times act in such a way as to promote and safeguard the well-being and interests of patients for whose care they are professionally accountable and ensure that by no action or omission on their part the patients' well being or safety is placed at risk.

Radiographers should introduce themselves to patients and should address patients in the appropriate manner.

Radiographers should ensure that patients are provided with information about their examination or treatment prior to, during and after the examination or treatment. They should ensure that patients leave the department understanding the appropriate follow-up procedure.

Patients must, wherever possible, have given informed consent, normally verbally but at times in writing, prior to any diagnostic imaging examination or radiotherapeutic procedure.

Patients have a right to refuse treatment or examination and this right should be respected. Where a patient refuses examination or treatment this should be reported to the referring clinician.

Refer to:

A guide to consent for examination or treatment – NHSME;
HC(90)22: A Guide to Consent for Examination or Treatment.

1.4   *Advocacy:* **Radiographers must, by virtue of their professional abilities, empower and enable patients such that they may make** their own decisions about the nature and progress of their examination or treatment.

At times patients' decisions may conflict with the beliefs or norms recognised by staff, but radiographers must support the patients' own decisions and act to promote those decisions.

2.   Professional integrity

2.1   *Personal Integrity:* The highest standards of personal integrity are expected; radiographers must comply with the laws of the country, state, province or territory of work.

Radiographers must avoid any abuse of the privileged relationship with patients and their relatives or the privileged access to their property.

2.2   *Discrimination:* Radiographers must ensure that their professional responsibilities and standards are not unduly influenced by considerations of age, disability, ethnicity, gender, nationality, party politics, race, religion, sexual preference, social or economic status, status in society or the nature of the patient's health problems.

2.3   *Toxic Substances:* Radiographers must not be under the influence of any toxic substance which impairs the performance of their duties.

2.4   *Personal Profit/Gain:* Radiographers must refuse to accept any gift, favour or hospitality which might be interpreted as seeking to exert undue influence to obtain early appointment or preferential treatment.

2.5   *Advertising:* Radiographers must avoid advertising or signing an advertisement using their professional qualification(s) to encourage the sale of commercial products.

3.   Professional relationships and responsibilities

3.1   *Professional Demeanour:* Radiographers should at all times act in such a manner as to justify public trust and confidence, to uphold and enhance the good standing and reputation of the profession, and to serve the public interest and the interests of the patients.

3.2   *Loyalty:* Radiographers should be loyal to fellow members of the profession and respect their dignity.

Loyalty within any profession cannot eventually override one's responsibility as a member of society to uphold its moral and legal obligations. Radiographers must ensure that unethical conduct and illegal professional activities are reported to their employer through their line manager.

It is the duty of members of the Society and College of Radiographers to uphold the professional standing of the organisation. This may require reference of unethical/illegal professional activities to the Society and College of Radiographers for consideration.

3.3 *Working Relationships:* **Radiographers should work in a collaborative and co-operative manner with others members of the healthcare team.**

3.4 *Conscientious Objection:* **Radiographers should make known to the employer any conscientious objection they hold which may be relevant to their professional practice.**

4. Professional standards

4.1 *Referral of Patients:* **Radiographers must only accept requests for examination or treatment which are properly authorised in accordance with established criteria and where those requests are for examinations or treatment that will be of benefit to the patient.**

Diagnostic imaging and interventional procedures should be performed and radiotherapy given only upon documented request by an approved referral source, e.g. registered medical and dental practitioners, chiropodists, podiatrists, chiropractors. The request must contain sufficient clinical information to justify the examination or treatment.

Radiographers may carry out alternative examinations or treatment where in their professional judgement the original request was inappropriate to the patient's condition and the clinical history provided.

Radiographers must refuse to carry out or assist with imaging and treatment procedures where, in their professional opinion, the risk to the patient is greater than the benefit to be obtained by the procedure.

4.2 *Safe Practice:* **All radiographers have a duty to ensure that a safe environment is maintained for staff, patients and visitors to the department.**

Radiographers should have due regard to the workload of, and pressures on, professional colleagues and subordinates and take appropriate action if these are seen to be such as to endanger safe standards of practice. Normally this will require issues to be raised with the employer through the line manager. However, in exceptional circumstances the Health and Safety Officer or Radiation Protection Supervisor should be informed.

Radiographers should have regard to physical working conditions and adequacy of resources and make known to the appropriate authority if these endanger safe standards of practice in any way.

If at any time guidelines, codes or policies are considered to impede the safe and effective performance of a radiographer's duties, proposals for change should be initiated through appropriate professional channels.

Radiographers are committed to keeping the radiation dose as low as reasonably practicable, consistent with diagnostic and treatment needs, and must apply this principle to any other imaging modality with which they work.

Radiographers must understand the implications of legislation relating to maintaining a safe environment, particularly Health and Safety legislation, Ionising Radiations Regulations legislation and approved codes of practice.

4.3 *Professional Development:* **Radiographers must take every reasonable opportunity to sustain and improve their knowledge and professional competence. They should promote the professional development and education of students and colleagues.**

As part of the professional development process radiographers should consider their personal and professional needs and translate these into realistic annual objectives and implementation plans which build into a professional portfolio.

Assurance of professional competence must be based on audit of professional practice activities which should be seen as a regular feature of radiographers' responsibilities.

Radiographers have a responsibility to assist in the professional development of other staff and students commensurate with their professional competence.

4.4 *Research:* **It is the duty of radiographers to develop the practice of radiography and as such engage in research and support the research of others.**

Radiographers should ensure that the results of all research undertaken by themselves or in collaboration with others are disseminated widely and that all people involved in the research are appropriately acknowledged.

4.5 *Role Development:* **Radiographers should develop their professional role. This may be done provided that they have been properly trained for the role development, there is an agreed written scheme of work and the employing authority has been informed in writing and assured of the radiographers' competence.**

Radiographers may provide a verbal comment on image appearance to the patient and should provide a written report to the referring clinician.

Radiographers may give injections and be involved in other clinical procedures.

Radiographers may administer radioactive products (radiopharmaceuticals) to patients when acting in accordance with directions of the local ARSAC licence holder (MARS 1978). The administration of such preparations must be in accordance with the said person's ARSAC licence scope and the said radioactive product must be administered only for the purpose so specified.

ARSAC   Administration of Radioactive Substances Advisory
             Committee.

MARS 1978   The Medicines (Administration of Radioactive Sub-
             stances) Regulations 1978, paragraph 2 (3).

Radiographers may undertake fluoroscopy where they believe it is in the best
interest of the patient. This is a matter for the professional judgement of the
radiographer.

NB: The notes above provide examples of professional role
     development activities. Radiographers are encouraged to
     initiate and participate in other professional role develop-
     ment activities.

4.6   *Legal Responsibility:* Radiographers are legally accountable for their
professional actions and for any negligence, whether by act or
omission or injury.

Index